Nutrition:
A Handbook for
Nurses

Edited by
Carolyn Best

Nutrition Nurse Specialist
Royal Hampshire County Hospital
Winchester

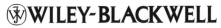

WILEY-BLACKWELL

A John Wiley & Sons, Ltd., Publication

This edition first published 2008
© 2008 John Wiley & Sons

Wiley-Blackwell is an imprint of John Wiley & Sons, formed by the merger of Wiley's
global Scientific, Technical and Medical business with Blackwell Publishing.

Registered office
John Wiley & Sons Ltd, The Atrium, Southern Gate, Chichester, West Sussex, PO19 8SQ,
United Kingdom

Editorial office
John Wiley & Sons Ltd, The Atrium, Southern Gate, Chichester, West Sussex, PO19 8SQ,
United Kingdom

For details of our global editorial offices, for customer services and for information about
how to apply for permission to reuse the copyright material in this book please see our
website at www.wiley.com/wiley-blackwell.

Library of Congress Cataloging-in-Publication Data

Nutrition : a handbook for nurses / edited by Carolyn Best.
p. ; cm.
Includes bibliographical references and index.
ISBN 978-0-470-06131-2 (pbk. : alk. paper)   1. Diet therapy – Handbooks,
manuals, etc.   2. Nutrition – Handbooks, manuals, etc.   3. Nursing – Handbooks,
manuals, etc.   I. Best, Carolyn.
[DNLM: 1. Nutrition Therapy – nursing.   WY 150 N9755 2008]
RT87.N87N868 2008
363.8 – dc22
2008013184

A catalogue record for this book is available from the British Library.

Set in 10 on 12 pt Palatino by SNP Best-set Typesetter Ltd., Hong Kong

Printed in Singapore by Markono Print Media Pte Ltd

1   2008

Nutrition:
A Handbook for
Nurses

Contents

Contributors

Carolyn Best
BSc (Hons), RGN, Dip HE
Nutrition Nurse Specialist

Helen Hitchings
BSc (Hons), RD, Dip ADP
Nutrition & Dietetic Services Manager

Harriet Gordon
MD, FRCP
Consultant Gastroenterologist

Joanna Boult
MPharm, DipClinPharm, MRPharmS (Gastroenterolgy)
Specialist Pharmacist

Preface

Good nutrition underpins good clinical care. Where a patient's nutritional intake is impaired over a period of time, nutritional deficiencies occur. The patient admitted to hospital may already be malnourished or have lost the desire or ability to eat, because of illness. This may be further compounded, following admission, by the need to place the patient 'nil by mouth' in preparation for procedures or operations. Failure to identify these problems and address the issues appropriately will lead to the patient's nutritional status being further compromised.

Nurses are the one group of healthcare professionals who provide 24-hour care for patients in a hospital setting and are therefore in an ideal position to identify nutritional problems and instigate initial care and onward referral. Unfortunately, nurses do not always recognise the important role they have to play in the patient's nutritional care.

This book aims to raise awareness and address some of the issues that nurses will encounter when caring for patients' nutritional needs in a hospital setting. It will also highlight the benefits that a hospital-based Nutrition Support Team can offer by providing a multidisciplinary approach to nutrition.

We write this book as an established, functioning Nutrition Support Team within a district general hospital that addresses patients' complex nutritional needs on a daily basis. We hope to educate but do not profess to provide all the answers to those difficult ethical issues or clinical decisions that may arise.

We hope you will find this book informative and easy to read and, although aimed primarily at nurses, hope it will be a reference guide for all clinical staff.

Carolyn Best
Nutrition Nurse Specialist

Introduction

This book aims to provide a comprehensive look at all aspects of nutrition, from roles and responsibilities to caring for a patient with specific nutritional needs.

The type and level of care required by patients will vary from one clinical setting to another. However, each will require specialist knowledge not only in terms of practical skills but also in terms of the assessment, monitoring and evaluation of the care provided. This book will present information that will enable the reader to update their knowledge and skills, which will hopefully equip them with the ability to offer a better standard of care to their patients. This book is structured to follow key issues with summary points and clinical case studies to be both an essential reference and educational tool.

We have planned the book to guide the reader through various stages of clinical nutrition, starting with Chapter 1 with a brief look into the national and European initiatives published since 1990 aimed at improving standards of nutritional care in primary and secondary care environments and influencing our clinical practice.

Chapter 2 looks at how malnutrition can develop, how to recognise the signs and makes recommendations for treatment. It also gives details on the consequences of poor, or non-, treatment of the condition and will look at the increasing need to recognise and manage malnutrition in obese patients.

Chapter 3 addresses the important issue of nutrition screening and identifies the difference between nutrition screening and assessment. We also look at when it is appropriate to refer the patient to a dietitian. Chapter 4 concentrates on the important but often unrecognised role that nurses have to play in ensuring that the patient receives the oral nutrition appropriate to their needs and the barriers that prevent this happening. We look at the initiatives that can assist in improving nutrient intake and make some suggestions for the education of nurses and carers.

Using a step-by-step approach, Chapter 5 takes the reader through the four stages of enteral nutrition support: ensuring the patient receives an appropriate oral diet, fortifying foods, nutritional supplements and enteral tube feeding. The section on enteral tube feeding provides information to enable the reader to appropriately care for the patient with an enteral feeding tube, looks at the issues around drug administration through feeding tubes, identifies potential complications and provides advice on how issues can be resolved. Chapter 6 moves on to the administration of parenteral nutrition, including clinical assessment of the patient, central line care, nutritional content of parenteral nutrition and care of the bag before use. Finally, this chapter looks at the role of non-medical prescribing in parenteral nutrition.

Chapter 7 looks at the process of starvation and the risk of refeeding syndrome when feeding is commenced, making recommendations to reduce the risks for staff at ward level.

In Chapter 8, we look at the legal and ethical issues that may arise when consideration is given to commencing nutrition support, an aspect of care that is becoming frequently discussed in the national press. We explore the decision-making process in the competent and incompetent patient, the use of advanced directives, feeding in dementia and persistent vegetative state and the difficulties that arise when considering withdrawing nutrition support.

Chapter 9 provides an insight into the setting-up of a hospital Nutrition Support Team and explores the benefits and difficulties that may be experienced by any district general hospital planning to establish such a team.

In Chapter 10, we look at the issues that may arise when discharging a patient from hospital to home with nutrition support, including the level of education and equipment required to ensure a safe transfer of care, the review process that should be undertaken to keep the patient stable at home and some of the potential problems that may arise.

In our final chapter, we present a number of case studies to demonstrate some of the issues we have had to face when considering options for nutritional care.

At the end of the book, the Glossary lists the various terms and acronyms used in the text, and in the field of nutrition.

Chapter 1

National and European Initiatives to Improve Standards of Nutritional Care

Carolyn Best

Introduction

In 1859, Florence Nightingale made the statement that 'thousands of patients are annually starved in the midst of plenty' (Tierney, 1996). Disturbingly, in the twenty-first century similar observations of patients in hospital are still being made.

Despite the clear indication that poor nutrition in hospital is not a new problem, little importance was attached to this aspect of health-care until the 1970s, when Butterworth (1974) in the United States of America discussed the issue of poor nutrition, and Bistrian *et al.* (1976) highlighted levels of poor nutrition of 44% or more. In 1977, Hill *et al.* examined surgical patients in Leeds, reporting that mal-nutrition and vitamin deficiency often went unrecognised and untreated by hospital staff and that few patients had even had their body weight measured. In spite of these research findings, 17 years later McWhirter and Pennington (1994) revealed that 200 out of 500 patients admitted to a hospital in Scotland were malnourished and that 75% of those patients followed lost further weight during their hospital stay.

In response to the recognition of the effect of poor nutrition on health, a number of policies, guidelines and resolutions were pub-lished towards the end of the twentieth and into this century in an attempt to address the problem.

To understand how these initiatives affect our daily working practice, and to set the scene for this book, it is important that we gain an insight into what each says. This chapter aims to give a brief outline of the aims of a number of UK and European initia-tives to improve the nutritional care of patients. The list discussed is by no means exhaustive, so apologies for any we have missed.

1

Where a report concerned discusses wider issues in relation to healthcare, we have highlighted those parts of it that refer to nutrition.

National and European initiatives 1990–2007

1990

Nutritional support in hospitals in the United Kingdom:
National survey 1988 (Payne-James et al., 1990)

Although the incidence of malnutrition in hospital patients had been recognised as a problem since the mid-1970s, until 1990 only two surveys had been undertaken in the United Kingdom that looked at the provision of nutrition support (Tredger *et al.*, 1981; Green *et al.*, 1987). Unfortunately, both of these studies only looked at nasogastric tube feeding.

The 1988 survey (Payne-James *et al.*, 1990) was undertaken to ascertain the level and type of nutrition support provided to the nutritionally compromised hospital patient in 206 districts in the United Kingdom. It looked at all the methods of nutrition support provided to patients. As dietitians were the only healthcare professionals solely working with patients with nutritional needs at the time, questionnaires were targeted at them. The survey reveals a wide variation in the provision of nutrition support throughout the country.

Its recommendations for the future of clinical nutrition support include:

- Each district (hospital) should have a group of people with an interest in clinical nutrition to monitor and advise on the care provided.
- The development of a national multidisciplinary group to advise, educate and promote the appropriate use of nutrition support and to encourage research into the field. This led to the development of the British Association for Parenteral and Enteral Nutrition (BAPEN).

1992

A Positive Approach to Nutrition as Treatment (Lennard-Jones, 1992)

This report was published to raise the awareness of healthcare professionals of the effects of poor nutrition and to improve the treatment of clinical malnutrition in hospital and at home through the development of local and national standards. This was the first document that set standards for nutrition in practice in the United Kingdom and stemmed from the results of the *Nutritional support in hospitals in the United Kingdom: National survey 1988* (Payne-James *et al.*, 1990).

1996

Standards and Guidelines for Nutritional Support of Patients in Hospital (Sizer, 1996)

This booklet, compiled by BAPEN, agreed national standards for the organisation and provision of nutrition support for patients in hospital.

The standards stipulate that there should be:

- a management policy within healthcare organisations stating that all patients receive adequate and appropriate nutrition support
- a functioning catering liaison group with representation from caterers, dietitians, nurses and doctors
- the development of a Nutrition Support Team to advise on all aspects of nutrition support
- the need to have organisation-wide policies in place for the provision of enteral and parenteral nutrition
- the provision of a continuing education programme addressing issues surrounding general nutrition and techniques of nutrition support for all staff involved in the clinical care of patients
- details on what care the patient can expect
- that there is a robust audit process in place.

1997

Hungry in Hospital? (Community Health Councils, 1997)

This briefing explores the issues around why some patients do not eat and drink enough when they are in hospital and who should be responsible for ensuring that patients' nutritional needs are met. It also makes recommendations to address the issues identified. It is based upon the experiences of a number of community health councils and the concerns relayed to them by families regarding the care their elderly relatives received in hospital. Much of the criticism for patients' poor food and fluid intake was aimed at nursing staff.

Eating Matters (Centre for Health Services Research, 1997)

Following the criticism aimed at nurses in the *Hungry in Hospital?* report, the Department of Health commissioned an education pack aimed at addressing nurses' understanding of the importance of nutrition and tackling practical issues to improve nutritional intake.

Eating Matters is the resource pack developed.

Its aims were to:

- help hospital staff meet patients' nutritional needs whilst they are in hospital
- offer practical solutions on how to audit and improve clinical practice
- provide a number of teaching aids and case studies.

Its chapters include:

- an overview of nutritional issues relating to the care of the patient in hospital
- educating ward staff
- issues around swallowing and the presentation of food
- fortifying foods
- auditing dietary care.

1998

Ethical and Legal Aspects of Clinical Hydration and Nutritional Support (Lennard-Jones, 1998)

This report highlights the ethical issues that surround any decision made for patients requiring nutrition support and offers guidance on appropriate action.

The report explores important issues, including:

- the impact of physical death and loss of personality
- defining the differences between withholding or withdrawing hydration or nutrition given through a feeding tube
- the difference between an act and an omission to act
- the rights of the competent patient
- protecting the rights of, and decision-making for, incompetent patients
- decision-making in infants, children and adolescents
- the right of the patient or family to demand fluid or nutrition via a tube.

1999

Current Perspectives on Enteral Nutrition in Adults (McAtear, 1999)

This document was released to provide up-to-date information on current practice in enteral feeding with the aim of assisting the development of local policies and procedures.

It addresses issues such as:

- why patients should be fed enterally
- which groups of patients should be fed enterally
- how a patient's nutritional requirements should be estimated
- route and tube options for enteral feeding
- the types of feed available for enteral feeding and when each should be used
- what monitoring should be undertaken
- possible complications that may arise and recommendations for management.

Managing Nutrition in Hospital: A Recipe for Quality
(Davis and Bristow, 1999)

This report focuses on the key organisational and management issues relating to food and feeding in hospital, from ward level upwards. The findings confirm the need for clear definitions of roles and responsibilities together with closer coordination of food provision and nutritional care at all levels within hospital Trusts.

Hospital Food as Treatment (Allison, 1999)

This report looks at inadequacies in the provision of hospital food and makes recommendations on how these issues could be addressed.

It addresses:

- the consequences of malnutrition
- common reasons why people don't eat in hospital
- the cost and prevalence of food wastage
- the level of nutrient consumption
- the screening, assessment and monitoring of patients
- improving the distribution and service of meals
- the nutritional requirements of patients
- staffing, staff training and education.

The report concludes that there is room for improvement in all aspects of care, from the nutrition screening of patients on admission to the development of appropriate menus and methods of serving food.

2000

Guidelines for Detection and Management of Malnutrition (British Association for Parenteral and Enteral Nutrition, 2000)

These guidelines discuss the development of a new screening tool for use in the detection and management of malnutrition in the community – the MAG tool. It includes explanations on how to use the tool and makes recommendations on areas for future audit/research.

Reducing Food Waste in the NHS (Department of Health, 2000a)

This publication promotes good practice in NHS hospitals to minimise food wastage.

It:

- considers who is responsible for controlling food waste
- identifies stages in the hospital food cycle
- makes recommendations for best practice.

It provides hospital managers and other professionals involved in the provision of food within hospitals with a guide highlighting where food waste occurs and how to control it. It also provides a tool for hospital caterers that encourages a multidisciplinary approach to monitoring and tackling food waste.

NHS Plan (Department of Health, 2000b)

The *NHS Plan* outlines the Department of Health vision of the future health service: a service 'designed around the patient'.

In relation to nutrition and food service, the *NHS Plan* states that by 2001 there would be a:

- 24-hour catering service available with a new NHS menu
- national franchise for NHS catering.

It also states that:

- housekeepers will be present on half of all wards by 2004
- dietitians will advise and check on the nutritional values of hospital food as part of the Performance Assessment Framework
- there will be a regular programme of unannounced inspections of the nutritional quality and presentation of hospital food.

2001

Essence of Care (Department of Health, 2001a)

This document arose from a commitment made in *Making a Difference: Strengthening the nursing, midwifery and health visiting contribution to health and healthcare* (Department of Health, 1999) to explore the benefits of benchmarking to help improve the quality of fundamental and essential aspects of care. It was designed to support the measures to improve quality set out in *A First-Class Service* (Department of Health, 1998) and help practitioners to take a structured approach to sharing and comparing practice, to identify best practice and to develop action plans to remedy poor practice.

Eight standards were agreed upon, of which the Food and Nutrition standard was the third. The Food and Nutrition standard was then broken down into 10 factors, each of which was to be audited and its performance measured:

1. screening and assessment to identify patients' nutritional needs
2. planning, implementation and evaluation of care assessments for those patients who require a nutrition assessment
3. a conducive environment (acceptable sights, smells and sounds)
4. assistance to eat and drink
5. obtaining food
6. food provided
7. food availability
8. food presentation
9. monitoring of food
10. eating to promote health

National Service Framework for Older People (Department of Health, 2001b)

In relation to nutrition, this framework states that 'nutritional risk screening should take place to identify those with characteristics of nutritional concern. For those at particular risk, a nutrition plan needs to be developed, appropriate food provided, food intake monitored and action taken if nutritional needs are not being met.'

Better Hospital Food Programme (NHS Estates, 2001)

The Better Hospital Food programme was designed to raise the profile of the quality of food offered to patients in NHS hospitals in England and to make effective changes to hospital food services nationwide. It followed the recommendations made in the *NHS Plan* (Department of Health, 2000b).

The Better Hospital Food programme's initial aims were to:

- produce a comprehensive range of tasty, nutritious and interesting recipes that every NHS hospital could use
- redesign hospital printed menus to make them more accessible and easier for the patient to understand
- introduce a 24-hour catering service to ensure food was available night and day
- ensure hot food was available in hospitals at lunchtimes and early-evening meals.

As a result of the work undertaken during this project, a number of initiatives were piloted and implemented, including:

- the National Dish Selector, containing over 300 recipes developed by a team of leading chefs for use in healthcare facilities
- the Flexi Menu, aimed at providing patients with a greater choice of meals
- protected mealtimes
- the provision of food 24 hours a day using:
  - light-bite hot meals, with dishes such as cottage pie and cod in parsley sauce
  - light refreshments provided through ward kitchens, such as tea or coffee with biscuits, cake or fresh fruit
  - snack boxes, containing sandwiches or cheese and crackers, a piece of cake or a biscuit, fruit and a drink.

Acute Hospital Portfolio: Review of National Findings – Catering (Audit Commission, 2001)

This review records the national results of an investigation of hospital catering carried out by the Audit Commission as part of its Acute Hospital Portfolio. It is based on data collected during 1999/2000 and involves the participation of most of the NHS hospitals in England and Wales.

The main areas reviewed in this report are:

- how patients' nutritional needs are identified and met
- the quality of the catering service provided and the relationship between quality and costs
- the actual expenditure on catering and the variation in spending between Trusts
- the management and control of costs
- the potential savings available from reducing food waste on wards.

In conclusion, the report states that:

1. There is scope for many Trusts to improve the quality of their catering service.
2. Patients' nutritional needs are not always identified or are not fulfilled, owing to limited menu choice, poor timeliness of meals or lack of assistance provided to eat.
3. More effective communication is required between the catering department and other staff to raise and then maintain the quality of the service delivered to patients.
4. Cost savings could be made through better pricing policies for non-patient services, reducing the waste of unserved meals.
5. Trusts need better information for decision-making and need effective mechanisms for ensuring that funds set aside for improving patient services are spent in this area and not redirected into subsidising non-patient services.
6. Patient satisfaction must be closely monitored to ensure that a tighter control of costs does not bring about a decline in service quality.

2002

Improving Health in Wales: Nutrition and Catering Framework
(Welsh Assembly Government, 2002)

This document sets a number of standards that Trusts in Wales are expected to meet, including that:

- All Trusts have nominated a single board member responsible for hospital nutrition and catering.

- Patients should expect:
  ○ a choice of meals
  ○ to be given assistance with eating their food if required
  ○ an uninterrupted period to eat their meal
  ○ meals and snacks to be available when mealtimes are missed.
- Trusts should develop a nutrition policy that clearly indicates the roles and responsibilities of staff regarding patient nutrition.
- Relevant procedures and protocols should be in place to cover issues such as:
  ○ screening/assessment of patients
  ○ ongoing nutrition assessments
  ○ measuring the intake of food and fluid
  ○ pre- and post-operative care and restriction of food and fluid intake.

Nutrition and Patients: A doctor's responsibility *(Royal College of Physicians, 2002)*

This report aims to highlight the role of a doctor in providing nutritional care for their patients in both a hospital and community setting and makes the following recommendations for medical staff.

All doctors should be aware:

- of a patient's nutrition problems and how to manage them
- that proper nutritional care is fundamental to good clinical practice.

Doctors should be responsible for ensuring that:

- adequate information concerning a patient's nutritional status is documented in the patient's clinical record
- appropriate action has been taken to deal with nutritional problems.

Doctors should play a role in:

- the multidisciplinary support required for patients with complicated malnutrition
- patients requiring long-term artificial enteral or parenteral nutrition.

Patient Environment Action Teams (PEAT) inspections
(Patient Environment Action Teams, 2002)

The PEAT programme was set up in 2000 to assess NHS hospitals. In 2002, its scope was extended to include assessments on the quality of food and food service. Under the programme, every in-patient health-care facility in England with more than 10 beds is assessed annually.

During a PEAT visit, meals and meals service are assessed and the organisation is given a rating based on a traffic-light system:

- **Green:** those organisations found to be providing high standards of food and food service that always, or almost always, met patients' needs and generally exceeds expectations. These organisations met the requirements of the Better Hospital Food programme.
- **Yellow:** those organisations found to be providing standards of food and food service that generally met patients' needs. However, these facilities had room for improvement in some areas.
- **Red:** those organisations found to be providing generally poor standards of food and food service that did not meet patients' needs and required urgent improvement.

PEAT results are given to the Healthcare Commission and results relating to food and food service are published on the Better Hospital Food website. Each year, the PEAT programme is adapted to reflect changing expectations within the NHS and to ensure that the results provide an accurate picture.

Promoting Nutrition for Older Adult In-patients in NHS Hospitals in Scotland (Scottish Executive, 2002)

This paper aims to provide a practical guide to clinical staff in implementing standards for nutritional care and focuses on:

- undertaking pre-admission assessments and nutrition screening for patients aged 65 years and over
- the importance of recognising the signs and symptoms of malnutrition
- menu design
- patient choice

- the roles of healthcare professionals in maintaining nutritional standards
- developing and undertaking training programmes.

Best Practice Statement: Nutrition Assessment and Referral in the Care of Adults in Hospital (Nursing and Midwifery Practice Development Unit, 2002)

The Nursing and Midwifery Practice Development Unit (NMPDU) is an organisation that identifies and disseminates best practice across Scotland. This paper highlights what actions constitute best practice in relation to:

- patients receiving appropriate nutritional care on admission to hospital
- nursing management of nutritional care
- screening and documentation
- criteria for nutritional referrals
- education and training.

2003

Care Homes for Older People: National Minimum Standards and the Care Homes Regulations 2001 (Department of Health, 2003)

This document, although dated 2001, was released in February 2003 and replaced earlier editions. It contains a statement of national minimum standards for older people in care homes. It covers all aspects of care, but Standard 15 relates specifically to nutrition, stating that: 'the registered person ensures that service users receive a varied, appealing, wholesome and nutritious diet, which is suited to assessed and recorded requirements, and that meals are taken in a congenial setting and at flexible times'.

In addition, it recommends that nursing homes should ensure that:

- care staff monitor the individual resident's food intake
- the availability, quality and style of presentation of food should be monitored
- residents should receive appropriate assistance at mealtimes
- the social aspects of food (its preparation, presentation and consumption) remain an important aspect of a resident's life wherever possible

- alternative ways of maintaining residents' involvement in food preparation and delivery are explored
- individuals' food preferences (personal and cultural/religious) are observed
- they do not make false claims that they can provide specialised diets (e.g. kosher or halal if they cannot observe all the requirements associated with those diets in terms of purchase, storage, preparation and cooking of the food).

Guidelines for Nutrition Screening (Kondrup et al., 2003)

This document sets out guidelines for hospitals and other healthcare organisations in the use of nutrition screening tools by proposing a set of standards for their use. It discusses what it calls 'the lack of a widely accepted screening system' and makes recommendations for practice.

It states how the effectiveness of a screening tool should be evaluated (Box 1.1) and that hospitals and healthcare organisations should have a policy and a specific set of protocols for identifying patients at nutritional risk, leading to the development of appropriate nutritional care plans.

Its suggested course of action includes:

- **Screening:** All patients should be screened on admission to hospital or other institutions. The outcome of screening must be linked to a defined course of action.

Box 1.1 Assessing the effectiveness of a screening tool (European Society for Parenteral and Enteral Nutrition)

- That the individual identified to be at risk is likely to obtain a health benefit from the intervention arising from the results of the screening (i.e. the predictive validity of the tool).
- The screening tool should have a high degree of content validity (i.e. it includes all relevant components of the problem it is meant to solve).
- It must have a high reliability (i.e. little interobserver variation).
- It must be a practical document that is simple to use.
- It should not contain irrelevant information.
- It should be linked to specified protocols for action, e.g.:
  - referral to a dietitian for those patients screened at risk
  - development of nutrition care plans.

Adapted from Kondrup *et al.*, 2003

- **Assessment:** A detailed examination of metabolic, nutritional or functional variables should be undertaken by an expert clinician, dietitian or nutrition nurse.
- **Monitoring and outcome:** The effectiveness of the care plan should be monitored by defined measurements and observations that will direct the nutritional care provided to the patient.
- **Communication:** Results of screening, assessment and nutritional care plans should be communicated to other healthcare professionals if the patient is transferred from one clinical area to another or from secondary to primary care (and vice versa).
- **Audit:** The need to develop a programme of audit to inform future policy decisions should be recognised.

Essence of Care: Patient-focused benchmarks for clinical governance (NHS Modernisation Agency, 2003)

This document updates the information released in 2001 and contains a toolkit for benchmarking the fundamentals of care.

It includes information on:

- the background to the *Essence of Care*
- a description of the benchmarking tool
- instructions on how to use the benchmarks
- the record forms for developing action and business plans
- the information to be measured to benchmark each standard.

The MUST report: Nutritional screening of adults: a multidisciplinary responsibility (Elia, 2003)

The *MUST* report provides evidence regarding the extent and effects of malnutrition in the United Kingdom, stating that:

- malnourished patients when discharged from hospital are two and a half times more likely to require healthcare at home
- underweight patients visit their GP more frequently and require more prescriptions
- malnourished individuals are more likely to need a longer stay in hospital.

It highlights the issue that the management and treatment of malnutrition often goes unrecognised and untreated in the United Kingdom and that £226 million could be saved each year in UK hospitals if malnourished patients were identified and treated appropriately. This report was used to launch the 'MUST' (Malnutrition Universal Screening Tool) as the first universal nutrition screening tool for adults to detect whether individuals have a low, medium or high risk of malnutrition, or are obese. It was the first nutrition screening tool designed for use in all healthcare settings and with all adult patients.

Standard for Hospital Food, Fluid and Nutritional Care in Hospitals (NHS Quality Improvement Scotland, 2003)

This report provides standards for the provision of food and the nutritional care of patients in hospital in Scotland and makes nutrition screening mandatory for every person admitted to hospital, acknowledging that the MUST screening tool is appropriate for this purpose.

Resolution ResAP (2003) 3: On food and nutritional care in hospitals (Council of Europe, 2003)

This resolution makes a number of recommendations that all governments of the member states, which includes the United Kingdom, should put into practice, including the need to draw up and implement national recommendations on food and nutritional care in hospitals.

2004

Patient Environment Action Teams (PEAT) inspections (Patient Environment Action Teams, 2004)

In 2004, a new system was used to represent the overall quality of food and food services in individual healthcare facilities. The assessment comprised a review of nine components relating to meals and their service and six Better Hospital Food requirements.

2005

Managing Food Waste in the NHS (NHS Estates, 2005)

This document aims to provide best practice guidance for modern matrons, doctors, dietitians, catering managers, ward housekeepers and ward-based teams and identifies reasons why food waste occurs in the ordering, distribution and service of food at ward level. It makes recommendations on how food waste can be managed in a cost-effective way. It was produced in response to the Audit Commission's *Acute Hospital Portfolio: Review of National Findings – Catering* (2001) and updates *Reducing Food Waste in the NHS* (Department of Health, 2000a) and provides guidance on:

• identifying the reasons for food wastage and definitions of food waste
• developing universally accepted tools to identify levels of food waste in order to enable effective comparisons between Trusts
• reducing the volume of food supplied or cooked but not served
• explaining why patients do not eat food served to them and developing appropriate action in response
• identifying the responsibilities for reducing food waste amongst members of the wider healthcare team.

The Cost of Disease-related Malnutrition in the UK and Economic Considerations for the Use of Oral Nutritional Supplements in Adults (British Association for Parenteral and Enteral Nutrition, 2005)

This report discusses the cost of malnutrition in the United Kingdom and details findings from a number of studies relating to the cost of using nutritional supplements in both the primary and secondary care settings and makes recommendations for future research.

2006

Nutrition Support in Adults: Oral nutrition support, enteral tube feeding and parenteral nutrition, Clinical Guideline 32 (National Institute for Health and Clinical Excellence, 2006)

These guidelines provide information to improve the practice of nutrition support in both hospital and community settings. The recommendations or guidelines are backed by evidence (where possible) or 'best practice' standards. Relevant information is provided to equip healthcare practitioners with the necessary information to recognise and treat poor nutrition using the most appropriate form of nutrition support for patients.

The guidelines cover information on:

• the prevalence of malnutrition
• the benefits of good nutrition
• who should be screened for malnutrition and when

- indications for nutrition support
- monitoring required for patients receiving nutrition support
- the administration of oral, enteral and parenteral nutrition
- appropriate access for enteral and parenteral nutrition
- supporting patients receiving enteral and parenteral nutrition support in the community.

Hungry to be Heard: The scandal of malnourished older people in hospital (Age Concern, 2006)

Age Concern uses this report to highlight the continuing problem of poor nutritional care for older people in hospital and calls for action from the NHS, Healthcare Commission and Department of Health.

It documents what it considers to be seven vital steps that need to be taken to end malnutrition in hospital:

1. Listening to older people, their relatives and carers.
2. Ensuring that all ward staff are 'food aware'.
3. Hospital staff must follow professional codes.
4. Patients are assessed for signs of malnourishment.
5. Protected mealtimes are introduced.
6. The 'red tray' system is implemented.
7. Volunteers are used to assist eating where appropriate.

Guidelines on Adult Enteral Nutrition (Lochs et al., 2006)

These are evidence-based guidelines on enteral nutrition. They discuss a wide range of issues, including:

- the patient journey
- ethical and legal aspects
- cardiology and pulmonology
- gastroenterology
- geriatrics
- hepatology
- wasting in HIV
- intensive care
- non-surgical oncology
- pancreas
- renal failure
- surgery and transplantation.

2007

Nutrition Now (Royal College of Nursing, 2007)

The Royal College of Nursing (RCN) developed this list of principles to guide nurses in their thinking regarding what can be done to improve the experience of the patient in relation to nutrition and hydration.

This initiative provides a framework and resources to educate nurses linking into relevant literature, as appropriate.

Subject areas covered include:

- malnutrition
- nutrition assessment
- nutrition in hospitals
- nutrition in the community
- older people
- patient information
- protected mealtimes
- case studies: to provide ideas on how nurses can improve nutrition in the area in which they work.

Improving Nutritional Care (Department of Health, 2007)

In response to the continuing concerns regarding patients/residents not receiving optimal nutritional care in the health and care systems, the Department of Health together with a number of other organisations, including the Food Standards Agency, BAPEN, the RCN and National Patient Safety Agency (NPSA), collaborated to make a number of recommendations for how, collectively, they and the government will tackle the issue.

The paper sets out the key priorities for action:

- To raise awareness of the link between nutrition and good health and that malnutrition can be prevented.
- To ensure that accessible guidance is available.
- To ensure that the most relevant guidance is appropriate and user-friendly.
- To encourage nutrition screening for all people using health and social care services, in particular those groups that are known to be vulnerable.
- To encourage provision and access to relevant training for front-line staff and managers on the importance of nutrition.
- To clarify standards and strengthen inspection and regulation.

Conclusion

A number of common threads can be seen running through the reports discussed.

You may recognise some that have filtered down to become accepted into everyday practice, for example protected mealtimes and the 'red tray' initiative. Other aspects, such as nutrition screening, continue to be an issue. There are no magic answers to these issues. The same problems are being addressed in hospitals throughout the United Kingdom.

It will be interesting to see what changes the future will bring and whether we are any better at caring for malnourished patients admitted to hospital.

References

Age Concern (2006) *Hungry to be Heard: The scandal of malnourished older people in hospital*, Age Concern, London.

Allison, S.P. (1999) *Hospital Food as Treatment: A report by a working party of the British Association for Parenteral and Enteral Nutrition*, BAPEN, Maidenhead.

Audit Commission (2001) *Acute Hospital Portfolio: Review of National Findings – Catering*, Audit Commission Publications, London.

Bistrian, B.R., Blackburn, G.L., Vitale, J. *et al.* (1976) Prevalence of malnutrition in general medical practices. *Journal of the American Medical Association* **235** (1515), 1567–70.

British Association for Parenteral and Enteral Nutrition (2000) *Guidelines for Detection and Management of Malnutrition: A report by the Malnutrition Advisory Group, a Standing Committee of BAPEN*, BAPEN, Maidenhead.

British Association for Parenteral and Enteral Nutrition (2005) *The Cost of Disease-related Malnutrition in the UK and Economic Considerations for the Use of Oral Nutritional Supplements in Adults: Executive summary*, BAPEN, Maidenhead.

Butterworth, C.E. (1974) The skeleton in the hospital closet. *Nutrition Today* **9** (2), 4–8.

Centre for Health Services Research (1997) *Eating Matters*, Centre for Health Services Research, University of Newcastle, Newcastle-upon-Tyne.

Community Health Councils (1997) *Hungry in Hospital? Association of Community Health: Health News Briefing*, Association of Health Councils for England and Wales, London.

Council of Europe (2003) *Resolution ResAP (2003) 3: On food and nutritional care in hospitals*, Council of Europe, Committee of Ministers, Strasbourg.

Davis, A.M., Bristow, A. (1999) *Managing Nutrition in Hospital: A Recipe for Quality*, Nuffield Trust Series No. 8, Nuffield Trust for Research and Policy Studies in Health Services, London.

Department of Health (1998) *A First-Class Service: Quality in the new NHS*, DH, London.
Department of Health (1999) *Making a Difference: Strengthening the nursing, midwifery and health visiting contribution to health and healthcare*, DH, London.
Department of Health (2000a) *Reducing Food Waste in the NHS*, Hospital Caterers Association in conjunction with NHS Estates, DH, London.
Department of Health (2000b) *NHS Plan: A Plan for Investment, A Plan for Reform*, DH, London.
Department of Health (2001a) *Essence of Care*, DH, London.
Department of Health (2001b) *National Service Framework for Older People*, DH, London.
Department of Health (2003) *Care Homes for Older People: National minimum standards and the care home regulations 2001*, DH, London.
Department of Health (2007) *Improving Nutritional Care: A joint action plan from the Department of Health and Nutrition Summit stakeholders*, DH, London.
Elia, M. (2003) *The MUST report: Nutritional screening of adults: a multidisciplinary responsibility: A report by the Malnutrition Advisory Group of the British Association for Parenteral and Enteral Nutrition*, BAPEN, Redditch.
Green, C., Tredger, J., Dickerson, J.W. (1987) Internal feeding: A survey to investigate current practices and attitudes of dietitians. *Human Nutrition Applied* **41A** (5), 360–3.
Hill, G.L., Blackett, R.L., Pickford, I. *et al.* (1977) Malnutrition in surgical patients: An unrecognised problem. *Lancet* **1** (8013), 689–92.
Kondrup, J., Allison, S.P., Elia, M. *et al.* (2003) European Society for Parenteral and Enteral Nutrition Guidelines for Nutrition Screening 2002. *Clinical Nutrition* **22** (4), 415–21.
Lennard-Jones, J.E. (1992) *A Positive Approach to Nutrition as Treatment*, King's Fund Centre, London.
Lennard-Jones, J.E. (1998) *Ethical and Legal Aspects of Clinical Hydration and Nutritional Support: A report for the British Association for Parenteral and Enteral Nutrition*, BAPEN, Maidenhead.
Lochs, H., Valentini, L., Schütz, T. *et al.* (2006) Guidelines on Adult Enteral Nutrition. *Clinical Nutrition* **25** (2), 177–360.
McAtear, C. (1999) *Current Perspectives on Enteral Nutrition in Adults: A report by a working party of the British Association for Parenteral and Enteral Nutrition*, BAPEN, Maidenhead.
McWhirter, J.P., Pennington, C.R. (1994) Incidence and recognition of malnutrition in hospital. *British Medical Journal* **308** (6934), 945–8.
National Institute for Health and Clinical Excellence (2006) *Nutrition Support in Adults: Oral nutrition support, enteral tube feeding and parenteral nutrition, Clinical Guideline 32*, NICE, London.
NHS Estates (2001) *Better Hospital Food Programme*, NHS Executive, London.
NHS Estates (2005) *Managing Food Waste in the NHS: Best practice guidance*, DH, London.
NHS Modernisation Agency (2003) *Essence of Care: Patient-focused benchmarks for clinical governance*, DH, London.

NHS Quality Improvement Scotland (2003) *Standard for Hospital Food, Fluid and Nutritional Care in Hospitals*, NHS QIS, Edinburgh.

Nursing and Midwifery Practice Development Unit (2002) *Best Practice Statement: Nutrition assessment and referral in the care of adults in hospital*, NMPDU, Edinburgh.

Patient Environment Action Teams (2002) Better Hospital Food, http://195.92.246.148/nhsestates/better_hospital_food/bhf_content/peat/2003_introduction.asp, accessed 16 November 2007.

Patient Environment Action Teams (2004) Better Hospital Food, http://195.92.246.148/nhsestates/better_hospital_food/bhf_content/peat/2004_introduction.asp, accessed 16 November 2007.

Payne-James, J., de Gara, C., Grimble *et al.* (1990) Nutritional support in hospitals in the United Kingdom: National survey 1988. *Health Trends* **22** (1), 9–13.

Royal College of Nursing (2007) *Nutrition Now*, RCN, London.

Royal College of Physicians (2002) *Nutrition and Patients: A doctor's responsibility*, RCP Publications, London.

Scottish Executive (2002) *Promoting Nutrition for Older Adult In-patients in NHS Hospitals in Scotland*, National Nursing, Midwifery and Health Visiting Advisory Committee, Edinburgh.

Sizer, T. (1996) *Standards and Guidelines for Nutritional Support of Patients in Hospitals: A report by a working party of the British Association for Parenteral and Enteral Nutrition*, BAPEN, Maidenhead.

Tierney, A. (1996) Undernutrition and elderly hospital patients: A review. *Journal of Advanced Nursing* **23** (2), 228–36.

Tredger, J., Bazin, C., Dickerson, J.W.T. (1981) Nasogastric tube feeding: A survey to investigate current practices and attitudes to dietitians. *Journal of Human Nutrition* **35** (118), 122.

Welsh Assembly Government (2002) *Improving Health in Wales: Nutrition and Catering Framework*. All-Wales Catering/Nutrition Group for the Welsh Assembly Government, Cardiff.

Chapter 2

Malnutrition

Harriet Gordon and Helen Hitchings

Introduction

Malnutrition is a common problem worldwide, and in developed countries it is associated particularly with poverty and alcoholism. It is also encountered among patients in hospital. Lean (2008) states that the number of malnourished patients being discharged from hospitals in England has increased by 85% in the past 10 years and that despite this increase malnutrition will be undiagnosed in up to 70% of patients.

Malnutrition to the layman usually means starvation, but the term has a much wider meaning encompassing the inadequacy of any nutrient in the diet. Whilst recognised in people with a limited or restricted food intake, it is also associated with excessive food intake. Patients with malnutrition may have evidence not only of protein-energy malnutrition but also of vitamin and mineral deficiencies, especially after major surgery or chronic illness.

What is malnutrition?

Malnutrition is caused by an inadequate availability of nutrients, because of either poor intake or deficiency as a result of disease. In developed countries, malnutrition is usually a consequence of disease. Attention should therefore be given to the treatment of the underlying disease, since this will often lead to a spontaneous improvement in nutritional status.

It is widely accepted that adequate nutrition plays an important role in maintaining optimal health. Malnutrition is the consequence of a nutritional intake that does not meet nutritional needs as a result of one or more of the following:

- decreased dietary intake
- increased nutritional requirements
- impaired ability to absorb or utilise nutrients.

Poor nutrition compromises immune function. Suppression of the immune system by malnutrition has been implicated as one of the major causes of complications in hospitalised patients (Ferguson *et al.*, 1999).

Primary malnutrition is seen in those who are dependent upon others for nourishment: infants, children, the elderly, the disabled, prisoners and the mentally ill are the most vulnerable groups. Secondary malnutrition is seen with any disease that disturbs appetite, digestion or the absorption of nutrients. Socioeconomic factors can profoundly influence nutritional status.

An individual's level of income also influences their food purchases and thus the quality of their diet. In general, the quality of the diet declines as income falls. At some point, the ability to purchase the foods required to meet nutritional needs is lost; an inadequate income puts an adequate diet out of reach. Low income affects not only the power to purchase foods but also the ability to shop for, store and cook them.

As discussed later in this chapter, you do not need to be thin to be malnourished. Inappropriate food choices may result in high-energy intakes, without the vitamins and minerals (micronutrients) required for health. For example, an over-reliance on fast foods and fizzy drinks may well provide adequate calories but suboptimal levels of vitamin C.

Hundreds of drugs interact with nutrients, making imbalances and deficiencies likely, especially in older people, who may be taking a number of different medications (polypharmacy). A number of drugs have side effects which will interfere with food intake, for example nausea, vomiting, constipation or diarrhoea.

Within the community, malnutrition has been described in up to 5% of the general population (Gregory *et al.*, 1990). Individuals may be eating well in the sense that they are meeting their calorie requirements, yet be malnourished owing to a poor choice of foods. Often during illness an individual's nutritional needs dramatically increase, owing to an increase in their metabolic rate and altered tissue metabolism. Within a hospital population, 10–44% of in-patients have been reported to have malnutrition (Bistrian *et al.*, 1976; Kelly *et al.*, 2000;

Box 2.1 Metabolic changes that occur following surgery or injury

Metabolic change	Consequence
Increased glycogenolysis	Leads to increased circulating blood glucose to be used as an energy substrate
Increased gluconeogenesis	Leads to increased circulating blood glucose to be used as an energy substrate
Increased lipolysis	Leads to increased free fatty acids, which are used to provide energy and increased glycerol that may be converted to glucose
Increased proteolysis	Leads to increased amino acids, which may be catabolised to provide energy or used for tissue synthesis and wound healing

McWhirter & Pennington, 1994) either contributing to their illness or as a consequence of it. In an elderly population, this increases to 29–61% (Corish & Kennedy, 2000). In the elderly a combination of factors can make malnutrition more common, for example physical frailty, deterioration of eyesight, hearing or dentition, poor mobility, social isolation, degenerative diseases, slight dementia, polypharmacy, relative poverty or an inability to purchase or prepare foods.

Malnutrition related to surgery or following severe injury occurs because of the extensive metabolic changes that accompany these events (Box 2.1).

These biochemical changes are mediated by the hormones cortisol, glucagon and catecholamine. They ensure survival in the short term, but at a price to the patient. Whereas loss of body fat may be acceptable and easily reversed, it is loss of muscle tissue that is of serious concern.

Those admitted to hospital with malnutrition have a significantly higher incidence of complications during treatment and a higher mortality rate than those who are well nourished on admission. Malnutrition has been shown to be an independent variable of length of stay, complication rate, mortality and cost (Hill *et al.*, 1977).

In 2006, the National Institute for Health and Clinical Excellence (NICE) issued guidelines on nutrition support for adults. The guidelines state that they aim 'to improve the practice of nutrition support by providing evidence and information for all healthcare professionals, patients and their carers so that malnutrition, whether in hospital or in the community, is recognised and treated by the best form of nutrition support at the appropriate time'.

Signs and consequences of malnutrition

Malnutrition has severe consequences, particularly during illness, where it can prolong the initial illness and a susceptibility to further problems. The effects of malnutrition if untreated are not limited to structural changes, such as a loss of body tissue, but can result in widespread physiological and functional effects as the body tries to adapt to the conditions of starvation and nutritional deficiencies.

These effects may include:

- impaired immune function, which increases risk of infection
- delayed wound healing
- increased risk of tissue breakdown and pressure ulcers
- muscle wasting and weakness, which can affect:
  - respiratory function
  - cardiac function
  - mobility
- altered structure of the small intestine (e.g. following surgery), which can result in malabsorption
- increased risk of post-operative complications
- apathy and depression
- general sense of weakness and illness.

When there is a reduction in nutritional intake, a number of changes take place. These can be seen in liver disease, starvation, intestinal disease, malabsorption, diarrhoea and psychiatric illness. This may also be observed in individuals who are repeatedly put 'nil by mouth' (NBM) prior to investigations or surgery. This may become a problem if it is repeated several times in a short period, for example if a planned operation or investigations are cancelled late in the day when the patient has been starved in anticipation of action, for example NBM from midnight for an operation planned for 2 p.m. that is then cancelled until the following day and the patient placed NBM from midnight the second night! Unfortunately, this is a scenario many of us will have witnessed.

During periods of reduced intake, the body initially supplements energy by releasing glycogen. Glycogen stores normally last for approximately 24 hours. Once all carbohydrate is utilised, the body turns its attentions to breaking down fats and proteins to release energy. The net effect of this will be a reduction in body mass and weight loss. Physiological mechanisms that conserve nutrients in the body are activated, and there is a reduction in the amount of work performed by the body. Spontaneous activity is usually reduced –

children no longer play or explore their environment, adults move as little as is necessary.

In malnutrition body composition alters. Initially, subcutaneous fat is lost, followed by muscle wasting. The more rapidly weight is lost, the more lean muscle tissue is lost in proportion to fat. Most tissues will contribute to weight loss, but they do not do so equally. Proportionately, body water increases, owing to oedema. This is due partially to the role albumin plays in its contribution to plasma osmotic pressure. If the serum albumin level drops to a very low level, oedema will develop.

Other causes of fluid retention or oedema include:

- medications (e.g. steroids)
- acute response to injury
- renal, cardiac and hepatic dysfunction.

The reduction in muscle mass leads to a reduction in respiratory function and the development of an ineffective cough. This in turn increases the risk of the patient developing more frequent chest infections that are of a longer duration. Cardiac muscle is impaired giving a poorer cardiac output, an increased risk of heart failure and cardiac fatigue. Heart rate is reduced.

Neurologically, the micronutrient deficiencies that occur as a consequence of malnutrition have severe consequences for all systems, for example the development of cardiac arrhythmia, apathy and depression.

Malnutrition is further compounded by a functional reduction in the gut. Intestinal motility is reduced and therefore intestinal transit time increased. The intestinal transit time is the time taken for a meal to travel from the mouth to the anus. This means more time for nutrients to be absorbed. There is a reduction in digestive enzyme activity leading to a reduction in the production of gastric acid, bile and pancreatic enzymes and the impairment of the gut lining. The cellular enzymes and transport systems for nutrient absorption are compromised, and the intestinal mucosa becomes flattened, further compounding the ability to absorb nutrients. Liver activity is down-regulated to such a point that fat export is impaired, resulting in the development of a fatty liver. Protein synthesis is reduced so that albumin and transferrin levels drop.

Routine biochemistry often includes total protein and albumin concentrations in a serum specimen, and globulin is often reported as the difference between the two. Changes in total protein concentration are common. A decreased total protein usually means the albumin concentration is low.

Albumin usually accounts for about 50% of the total hepatic protein production. It has a biological half-life in plasma of about 20 days. There are three main reasons for the occurrence of a low plasma albumin concentration:

- **Decreased synthesis:** This may be due to malnutrition or malabsorption. Decreased synthesis is also a feature of advanced chronic liver disease.
- **Abnormal distribution or dilution:** Hypoalbuminaemia can be induced by overhydration or if there is increased capillary permeability, as occurs in septicaemia.
- **Abnormal excretion or degradation:** The causes include nephrotic syndrome, protein-losing enteropathies, burns, haemorrhage and catabolic states.

Serum albumin measurements are often used to monitor a patient's response to nutrition support; however, they are unreliable and insensitive for this purpose and should not be used. Albumin is of limited value in monitoring nutritional status because of its long half-life, and because of its distribution in extracellular fluid. It is more a marker of illness and wellness than an absolute marker for nutrition, particularly when used in conjunction with C-reactive protein (CRP) level. CRP is involved in the immune and acute phase response, and is raised in illness, especially infection.

The kidney has a restricted ability to concentrate and dilute. Renal function is therefore reduced with poor-quality urine.

The basal metabolic rate drops and biochemically the cell membrane sodium-potassium pump rate drops, resulting in a rise in total body sodium and a reduction in potassium. Once feeding restarts and the pump becomes more active, there can be a catastrophic fall in intracellular potassium, a consequence of the development of 're-feeding syndrome'.

Temperature regulation becomes altered in malnutrition, and the individual becomes poikilothermic (meaning the body temperature fluctuates in response to temperature changes in the environment). In a cold situation, individuals become hypothermic, and hypoglycaemia may develop. Malnourished individuals do not shiver: this would increase energy expenditure, and so careful monitoring of vital signs in such patients becomes extremely important. Similarly, in the heat, rather than sweating, the body temperature rises. This may be a presenting feature of malnutrition in the elderly.

The body's stress response to starvation and malnutrition is seen hormonally with an increase in cortisol, a blunting of insulin and a reduction in thyroxine, which can all reduce metabolic rate in an attempt to conserve energy.

One of the most-studied consequences of malnutrition is that relating to the immune system. The immune system is susceptible to alterations in protein status; it is dependent on amino acids and proteins, such as immunoglobulins and cytokines, therefore protein-energy malnutrition results in a reduction in immunity and an increased risk of infections (Bistrian *et al.*, 1976).

Malnourished surgical patients have a delayed recovery time, with a greater morbidity and mortality, particularly from wound infections, compared to well-nourished patients (Correia & Waitzberg, 2003).

Specific deficiencies

Malnutrition may be due to:

• inadequate energy intake
• inadequate protein intake
• inadequate vitamins or minerals.

Protein-energy malnutrition is the inadequate intake of protein, mainly seen in developing countries. Kwashiorkor is the name given to malnutrition resulting from protein deficiency, while marasmus is a deficiency of both protein and energy.

Kwashiorkor results in:

• muscle wasting
• a low serum albumin resulting in peripheral oedema (which may make the muscle wasting less obvious)
• fatty liver with hepatomegaly.

There is a reduction in immunity and infections may also be present. It is usually seen in children and so there is also growth retardation. All these features are reversible with an adequate protein intake.

Marasmus is due to both protein and energy deficiencies, which are characterised by the classic features of starvation, including:

• growth reduction
• absence of body fat
• muscle wasting.

Within a hospital setting in developed countries, protein-energy malnutrition may be due to poor nutritional intake in alcohol misusers or in those suffering from anorexia nervosa. It may be seen in some conditions, because of an inability either to adequately absorb nutrients, such as with Coeliac disease, or to utilise that which is absorbed, such as in cirrhosis. Protein loss can occur following excessive losses of protein in the urine, such as in nephrotic syndrome or other renal disorders, and in acute surgical trauma or burns, owing to catabolism. Finally, increased utilisation and therefore protein intake requirements occur in fevers and hyperthyroidism.

* As numerous reports show (Community Health Councils, 1997; Department of Health, 2001; Age Concern, 2006), malnutrition can occur in the hospital setting, particularly in older patients who are in hospital for a number of weeks, owing to poor attention to their nutritional needs, for example lack of nutrition screening, food left out of the patient's reach, not providing appropriate assistance to eat or drink etc. *

Death from protein-energy malnutrition and other nutritional deficiencies occurs within 60 to 70 days of total starvation in normal-weight adults, but over a shorter period of time in those who are already malnourished. Depletion of nutrient stores also occurs more rapidly in the 'metabolically stressed patient'.

Specific vitamin and mineral deficiencies

Vitamin A

The absorption of vitamin A is related to fat absorption in the gut, and requires protein for synthesis. Therefore, a deficiency of fat, protein or a gut-related illness can result in vitamin A deficiency. Deficiency results in growth reduction and visual problems. Xerophthalmia may occur in vitamin A deficiency and is characterised by conjunctivitis, abnormal and severe dryness of the surface of the cornea and conjunctiva. Bitot's spots (white, soft deposits on the conjunctiva) and night blindness may also occur. Where a deficiency exists, there may be a reduction in immunity. This reduction was demonstrated to be reversible in 1932 where a daily dose of cod liver oil (which contains vitamin A) was given to children suffering with measles to boost their immunity. It resulted in a decrease in mortality from 8.7% to 3.7% (Ellison, 1932).

In a previously adequately nourished individual, there are usually enough stores of vitamin A within the liver to last approximately nine months, so it is not unusual for patients to present late in chronic illness.

Good dietary sources of vitamin A (and beta-carotene, a precursor to vitamin A) include:

- carrots
- oily fish
- liver and liver products
- fortified margarine and fat spreads
- fish liver oils
- dairy products (milk, cheese, cream and butter)
- egg yolks
- peaches, apricots and mangoes
- tomatoes and red peppers
- dark-green leafy vegetables (such as spinach).

Vitamin B1 (thiamine) deficiency

Vitamin B1 deficiency may be seen in individuals who abuse alcohol as, although it is present in many foodstuffs, vitamin B1 is not present in alcohol. In addition, the body does not store vitamin B1, as it is a water-soluble vitamin. Thiamine is mainly required during the metabolism of carbohydrates, fat and alcohol. Diets high in carbohydrate require more thiamine than diets high in fat. The deficiency is commonly known as beriberi. 'Dry beriberi' refers to the development of neurological problems, such as Wernicke's encephalopathy (ataxia, confusion, nystagmus and sixth cranial nerve palsy), peripheral and motor neuropathy. 'Wet beriberi' refers to the development of neurological problems with additional heart failure. The problems are reversible if sufficient thiamine is given, intravenously if necessary.

Sources of thiamine

Thiamine is not evenly distributed in cereal grains – most of it is present in the outer 'germ' layer. Hence, in the United Kingdom all flour other than wholemeal flour is required by law to be fortified with thiamine.

Other good sources include:

- yeast and yeast extract
- wholegrain cereal foods
- pork
- nuts
- pulses.

Many breakfast cereals are fortified with thiamine.

Vitamin B2 (riboflavin)

Vitamin B2 is water-soluble and is found in small amounts in many foods. However, levels rapidly decrease under serious illness or with the intake of some drugs, for example amitriptyline, imipramine, chlorpromazine or oral contraceptives.

A deficiency of riboflavin results in lesions on the mucocutaneous surfaces of the mouth (angular stomatitis, atrophic lingual papillae and magenta tongue), cracked, bleeding lips and glossitis. Itchy perineum and hair loss may be seen. There may also be neurological sequelae with photophobia and ataxia.

Riboflavin deficiency is often accompanied by iron deficiency – possibly as a result of impaired absorption.

Good dietary sources of riboflavin include:

- yeast and yeast extract
- liver and offal meats
- green, leafy vegetables
- eggs
- milk and dairy products and cereals and cereal products.

Folic acid

Folic acid is the parent molecule of a large number of derivatives collectively known as 'folates'. In deficiency states, it causes megaloblastic anaemia, atrophic tongue and growth retardation.

Deficiency is most likely to occur as a result of:

- **Malabsorption** (e.g. in Coeliac disease): The use of certain drugs interferes with folic acid metabolism (notably methotrexate to treat rheumatoid arthritis and anticonvulsants used in the treatment of epilepsy).
- **Cell proliferation:** Some disease states can cause an increase in cell proliferation (e.g. leukaemia).

Good dietary sources of folates include:

- liver
- green vegetables
- yeast extract
- pulses
- some fruits (oranges and orange juice).

There has been much debate regarding the fortification of all flour in the United Kingdom with folate. It is common practice in a number of other countries, including the United States of America and Canada.

This is primarily because of the role of folic acid in preventing neural tube defects in early pregnancy. To date, fortification is not common practice within the United Kingdom as there is some concern that folate supplementation can mask vitamin B12 deficiency in the elderly.

Vitamin C (ascorbic acid)

Vitamin C is water-soluble and easily destroyed in cooking. It is biochemically active in collagen synthesis, iron absorption and in immunologic function. Therefore, not surprisingly, a deficiency in vitamin C, better known as 'scurvy', is characterised by swollen, bleeding gums, wiry hair, anaemia and a predisposition to infections, and easy bruising. Overt scurvy is rarely seen in the United Kingdom; however, people with poor diets devoid of fresh food, and those with increased vitamin C requirements, such as cigarette smokers or post-operative patients, are likely to have suboptimal levels.

Owing to its role in collagen synthesis, adequate vitamin C is essential for wound healing.

Good dietary sources of vitamin C include:

- fruits and fruit juices (particularly citrus fruits, strawberries, kiwi fruit, berries, currants and guava)
- some green vegetables (such as green peppers, broccoli, cabbage and spring greens); however, significant losses can occur during storage and cooking.

Zinc

A deficiency in zinc may occur in patients who require long-term administration of parenteral or enteral feeding, if they have high requirements, with only standard amounts being provided. There are very small body stores of zinc; so problems can arise if it is not present within the diet on a regular basis.

Conditions which predispose people to zinc deficiency are related to:

- reduced intake (perhaps associated with an eating disorder)
- reduced absorption/bioavailability (owing to an inhibitor, such as a high-phytate diet)
- increased losses (such as in diarrhoea or excessive vomiting)
- increased requirement associated with growth (also in pregnancy/lactation)
- and are secondary to conditions such as alcoholism.

Deficiency results in poor hair quality and hair loss. Changes in the skin result in crusty lesions around the nose and mouth, followed by fingers, toes and the perineal area. The patient may go on to develop diarrhoea, mental confusion and depression. There is also an increased susceptibility to infections, as zinc has a critical role in immunocompetence. Zinc deficiency in childhood results in stunted growth. Zinc is also thought to play a role in taste acuity, and a loss of taste (hypogeusia) may result from zinc deficiency.

Zinc has a critical role in protein synthesis and in structural proteins; hence, a deficiency may impair wound healing. It has been postulated that zinc is related to appetite, as it is not unusual to have a loss of appetite with subclinical zinc deficiency.

Good dietary sources of zinc include:

- red meat
- fish and shellfish
- milk and milk products
- poultry
- eggs
- other sources of zinc include bread and cereal products, green, leafy vegetables and pulses, although these all have a lower bioavailability.

Iron

Iron is an essential component of haemoglobin and myoglobin, with its major function being that of carrying oxygen. Many enzymes contain or require iron, and it is required for many metabolic processes.

In contrast to other minerals, no mechanism exists in the body to excrete iron, therefore body levels of iron are regulated by absorption.

Iron deficiency results in a reduced ability to transport oxygen around the body. This can have many harmful effects on cardiovascular and respiratory systems, brain and muscle function, and wound healing.

Both a deficiency and excess of iron are associated with an increased susceptibility to infection. Iron deficiency, with or without anaemia, results in a wide range of defects in immune function.

Good dietary sources of iron include:

- red meat, liver and offal
- poultry and fish (contain smaller amounts)

- cereal products and fortified breakfast cereals; these can contribute significant amounts of non-haem iron, but this is less well absorbed than iron from meat products (haem iron).

Other good sources of non-haem iron include green leafy vegetables, dried fruit, pulses, nuts and seeds.

Having a good source of vitamin C (for example fruit or fruit juice) with foods that contain non-haem iron can enhance the absorption of iron. Tannins and phytates can inhibit the absorption of non-haem iron.

Iron and zinc compete for absorption, which is why it can be a disadvantage for people to self-supplement with either of these nutrients unless there is a proven deficiency and they are under medical supervision.

Management of malnutrition

Malnutrition within a hospital has repeatedly been shown to be under recognised, and inadequately treated (McWhirter & Pennington, 1994; Stratton *et al.*, 2003, 2004). Hospitalised patients are more likely to be malnourished than the general population, and yet the provision of appropriate nutrition although vital to support their recovery is not always available at the point of need. Consequently, it is essential to ensure that medical and financial resources are made available to support nutritional care and the importance of nutrition is recognised to ensure the patient receives the food they require.

In the 1990s, the importance of developing standards for nutritional care in hospital began to be recognised (Lennard-Jones, 1992; Allison, 1999) and the need for a multidisciplinary and hospital-wide approach to ensure the optimal management of nutrition (Silk, 1994). Good communication between the different professions involved in patient care is essential to ensure the provision of appropriate nutrition.

Those patients who are malnourished, or at risk of malnutrition, need to be identified so that a plan of care can be developed and implemented.

NICE guidelines (2006) recommend that this includes patients who present with:

- a body mass index (BMI) of less than $18.5 \, \text{kg/m}^2$, or
- have recently lost more than 10% of their body weight unintentionally, or
- have a BMI of less than $20 \, \text{kg/m}^2$, and 5% recent weight loss

or:

- if the patient has not eaten for five days and is unlikely to eat for at least the next five days
- has large nutritional losses, is highly catabolic or has a poor absorptive capacity.

In either of these groups, the most appropriate form of nutrition support, whether oral, enteral or parenteral, should be considered.

During illness, or following surgery, it is not uncommon for the appetite to become depressed. Therefore, the appetite can usually be used as an indicator of progress. Anorexia is a warning that something is wrong metabolically. The return of appetite means that infections are under control and there is no major electrolyte imbalance or deficiency.

An appropriately nourished individual is well equipped to resist disease, recover from illness, reach an optimal fitness level and enjoy a better quality of life.

Nutrition support

Despite help with and support to eat food whilst in hospital, there will always be a number of patients who, owing to their underlying illness or condition, will require further nutrition support. This may be either enterally (using supplemented diet, sip feeds or liquid nutrition) or intravenously (using parenteral nutrition). Therapeutic feeding will require appropriate line access, whether by a fine-bore nasogastric/nasojejunal feeding tube, percutaneous endoscopic gastrostomy (PEG), or jejunostomy, or by a central catheter for parenteral nutrition (PN).

The nurse's role

Nurses have a vital role in assessing and monitoring a patient's nutritional status. Nutrition screening is mandatory in hospitals in Scotland (NHS Quality Improvement Scotland, 2003) but not in England and Wales. It is, however, considered best practice that all patients in England and Wales be nutritionally screened on admission to hospital. Nurses weigh and measure patients, which enables them to calculate a patient's BMI. They are also in a key position to ask questions regarding recent weight loss, and appetite and dietary changes.

In an attempt to formalise nutrition screening, Elia (2003) launched the validated Malnutrition Universal Screening Tool, or MUST. The

MUST has been shown to give reproducible results in a range of settings.

During a patient's stay in hospital, repeated weights need to be taken, and clearly documented, at regular intervals as weight loss within hospital is common: 78% of the patients followed were found to have lost weight in the study undertaken in a hospital in the United Kingdom by McWhirter and Pennington (1994). The frequency of weight measurements will depend upon the patient's illness and the acuity of that illness.

Food- and fluid-intake charts and nutritional care plans frequently need to be implemented by nursing or care staff, as they are the healthcare professionals in most frequent contact with the patient, and are therefore best placed to notice when someone is failing to eat an adequate amount.

The nurse is also responsible for facilitating adequate food suitable to the patient, and in a manner that they can take it. It may be necessary to refer to a dietitian or speech and language therapist to achieve this.

Catering staff

Food needs to be accessible, palatable and nutritious. To achieve this, there needs to be an effective communication channel between Trust management, hospital chefs, dietetic departments, clinical areas and patients so that appropriate meals can be provided 24 hours a day to those that require them.

Hospital catering is often seen as a Cinderella service, given little respect, only contacted when there is a problem with a meal and often not considered to be involved in patient care, but it has a vital role to play in providing adequate and appealing nutrition for patients – often on a budget of less than £2–£2.50 per day per patient.

Dietitians

Dietitians frequently work with catering staff at a strategic level to ensure that the meals provided are healthy and well balanced. Largely, this may be achieved in the planning, monitoring and quality control of menus. In selected cases, following referral by a nurse, doctor or speech and language therapist, special diets or support may be required.

Referral to a dietitian for those at risk, i.e. with a BMI <18.5 kg/m^2, is essential and should be made as soon as possible once all criteria for referral have been met, i.e. the patient has been nutritionally screened and action plans within the screening tool have been implemented by nursing staff. Referral to the dietitian is also recommended for those patients who present with specific conditions, such as renal or liver failure, or a non-functioning gut.

Dietitians can provide a more formal assessment of nutrition assessment and may use anthropometric measurements to determine, for example, the triceps' skin-fold thickness, indicating fat storage, while the mid-arm muscle circumference indicates muscle mass.

Medical staff

The role of the medical practitioner is to recognise the signs of malnutrition through clinical assessment and thorough history-taking and to liaise with other healthcare professionals to organise referrals for further assessment, for example to speech and language therapists, dietitians, clinical psychologists, occupational therapists and the Nutrition Support Team.

Recognising and managing malnutrition in obese patients

Obesity does not preclude patients from developing malnutrition, though it may be a natural reaction to think it should. Obese individuals do not usually appear malnourished. The increasing prevalence of obesity in the community suggests that an increasing number of patients admitted to hospital will be obese. Increased morbidity has been reported in the injured obese patient; this may be related to poor nutrition support. If an obese individual has been trying to lose weight prior to their admission to hospital, this should be an indication that they may be at risk of malnutrition. It can be difficult to consume all the essential nutrients (vitamins and minerals) together with adequate protein in an energy-restricted diet. It can also be difficult to consume all the essential nutrients if the diet mainly consists of high-energy, low-nutrient foods – such as fizzy drinks, sweets and cakes – rich in fats, oils and sugar. An excess of energy is consumed; however, the diet may still be deficient in essential nutrients such as minerals, vitamins and essential fatty acids. In such cases, individuals are consuming adequate energy, although the quality of their diet is poor. This phenomenon has been termed 'modern malnutrition'.

Although obesity may give an increased chance of survival in situations of starvation, it does not seem to confer the same advantage following injury, when metabolic response is exaggerated in these individuals (Elia, 2003).

A thorough nutrition screening (and, where required, assessment) process should identify obese individuals who are at risk nutritionally, and allow an appropriate nutritional care plan to be implemented accordingly, as should be the case in all patients, whether obese or not. Historically, screening tools simply relying on BMI as an indicator for nutrition support need would classify overweight or obese patients as at minimal or no nutritional risk. Often the protocol for this would mean they are not re-screened. As is the case of patients who are not obese, this can result in increased length of hospital stay, increased length of rehabilitation and increased morbidity. It is likely that the identification of potential risk in obese injured patients goes beyond the measurement of indices such as BMI and percentage weight loss (Davidson & Smith, 2004).

Conclusion

It is important to remember that screening will only indicate nutritional risk, not actual nutritional status. The screening process is not a means to an end; it is a way of informing the healthcare practitioner whether a more objective nutrition assessment is required. In hospitals where a thorough nutrition screening process is undertaken on admission and the use of a multidisciplinary approach to nutrition is used, the effects of malnutrition can be minimised. It is important to remember that malnutrition is both a cause and a consequence of ill health, and that it is surprisingly common in the United Kingdom (National Institute for Health and Clinical Excellence, 2006).

References

Age Concern (2006) *Hungry to be Heard: The scandal of malnourished older people in hospital*, Age Concern, London.

Allison, S. (1999) *Hospital Food as Treatment: A report by a working party of the British Association for Parenteral and Enteral Nutrition*, BAPEN, Maidenhead.

Bistrian, B.R., Blackburn, G.L., Vitale, J. *et al.* (1976) Prevalence of malnutrition in general medical practices. *Journal of the American Medical Association* **235** (1515), 1567–70.

Community Health Councils (1997) *Hungry in Hospital? Association of Community Health: Health News Briefing.* Association of Health Councils for England and Wales, London.

Corish, C.A., Kennedy, N.P. (2000) Protein-energy under nutrition in hospital in-patients. *British Journal of Nutrition* **83** (6), 575–91.

Correia, M.I., Waitzberg, D.L. (2003) The impact of malnutrition on morbidity, mortality, length of hospital stay and costs evaluated through a multivariate model analysis. *Clinical Nutrition* **22** (3), 235–9.

Davidson, I., Smith, S. (2004) Nutritional screening: Pitfalls of nutritional screening in the injured obese patient. *Proceedings of the Nutrition Society* **63** (3), 421–5.

Department of Health (2001) *National Service Framework for Older People*, DH, London.

Elia, M. (2003) *The MUST report: nutritional screening of adults: a multidisciplinary responsibility. A report by the Malnutrition Advisory Group of the British Association for Parenteral and Enteral Nutrition*, BAPEN, Redditch.

Ellison, J.B. (1932) Intensive vitamin therapy in measles. *British Medical Journal* **11**, 708–11.

Ferguson, M., Capra, S., Bauer, J., Banks, M. (1999) Development of a valid and reliable malnutrition screening tool for adult acute hospital patients. *Nutrition* **15** (6), 458–64.

Gregory, J., Foster, K., Tyler, H., Wiseman, M. (1990) *The Dietary and Nutritional Survey of British Adults*, Office of Population Censuses and Surveys, Her Majesty's Stationery Office, London.

Hill, G.L., Blackett, R.L., Pickford, I. *et al.* (1977) Malnutrition in surgical patients: An unrecognised problem. *Lancet* **1** (8013), 689–92.

Kelly, I.E., Tessier, S., Cahill, A. *et al.* (2000) Still hungry in hospital: Identifying malnutrition in acute hospital admissions. *Quarterly Journal of Medicine* **93**, 93–8.

Lean, M. (2008) Malnutrition in hospital: Still common because screening tools are underused and poorly enforced. *British Medical Journal* **336**, 290.

Lennard-Jones, J.E. (1992) *A Positive Approach to Nutrition as Treatment*, King's Fund Centre, London.

McWhirter, J.P., Pennington, C.R. (1994) Incidence and recognition of malnutrition in hospital. *British Medical Journal* **308**, 945–8.

National Institute for Health and Clinical Excellence (2006) *Nutrition Support in Adults: Oral nutrition support, enteral tube feeding and parenteral nutrition, Clinical Guideline 32*, NICE, London.

NHS Quality Improvement Scotland (2003) *Standard for Hospital Food, Fluid and Nutritional Care in Hospitals*, NHS QIS, Edinburgh.

Silk, D.B.A. (1994) *Organisation of Nutritional Support in Hospitals: Nutrition steering committee and nutrition support teams – needs, structure and roles. A report by a working party of the British Association for Parenteral and Enteral Nutrition*, BAPEN, Maidenhead.

Stratton, R.J., Green, C.J., Elia, M. (2003) *Disease-Related Malnutrition: an Evidence Based Approach to Treatment*, CABI Publishing, Oxford.

Stratton, R.J., Hackston, A., Longmore, D. *et al.* (2004) Malnutrition in hospital out-patients and in-patients: Prevalence, concurrent validity and ease of use of the 'malnutrition universal screening tool' ('MUST') for adults. *British Journal of Nutrition* **92** (5), 799–808.

Chapter 3

Nutrition Screening and Assessment

Helen Hitchings

Introduction

As discussed in the previous chapter, malnutrition is a common problem. If left untreated, it leads to increased morbidity and mortality. Appropriate nutrition screening and assessment are vital in the early detection and treatment of poor nutritional status. Nutrition screening should be a quick, simple procedure undertaken within 24 hours of admission, usually by nursing staff. The nurse is the one healthcare professional in closest contact with the patient over a 24-hour period and should therefore have more information about the patient's eating habits and nutritional status. It makes sense that the responsibility for nutrition screening lies with them. A nutrition assessment is a more in-depth process which should be determined by the results of nutrition screening, and if necessary undertaken by a dietitian or Nutrition Support Team.

Nutrition screening

Nutrition screening is one of the processes used to identify those patients at risk of malnutrition, so that appropriate nutritional care plans can be instigated in a timely fashion.

Numerous reports recommend the use of nutrition screening for all patients on admission to hospital, including Allison (1999), Department of Health (2001) and National Institute for Health and Clinical Excellence (NICE; 2006).

NICE (2006) recommends that all hospital in-patients should be screened on admission and all out-patients at their first attendance. It also recommends that screening should be a routine and regular undertaking in primary care settings and in residential or nursing homes. Despite the more extensive use recommended by NICE, nutrition screening is probably more commonly associated with admission to hospital.

In 2007, the British Association for Parenteral and Enteral Nutrition (BAPEN; 2007) facilitated a nationwide screening week to look at the prevalence of malnutrition on admission to hospital. The survey identified that more than one in four adults admitted to hospital, mental units or care homes were at risk of malnutrition and urged all such institutions to implement nutrition screening on admission to ensure that patients at risk of malnutrition are identified and that a nutritional care plan is provided for them.

A basic nutrition screen may include some or all of the following:

- A review of the patient's diet, drug and medical history.
- Weighing the patient on admission, recording height measurements and determining weight for height, i.e. calculating body mass index (BMI).
- History of recent weight loss.
- Eyeball assessment, i.e. look at the person for obvious signs of weight loss or malnutrition.
- Looking at food and fluid intake.

Screening is the responsibility of all members of the multidisciplinary team, and could be undertaken by nurses, doctors, dietitians or other healthcare professionals. Where screening is difficult, for example where the patient is a poor historian or is unconscious, alternative methods of obtaining information should be sought from family or carers.

Screening would usually precede nutrition assessment, with those individuals identified at high risk of becoming malnourished being referred to a dietitian for a more thorough nutrition assessment.

It is important to recognise that the screening process should not be viewed as a one-off event. As part of the monitoring process, screening should be repeated at regular intervals. NICE (2006) recommends that screening be repeated weekly for in-patients, and where there is clinical concern for out-patients.

It is good practice to have a robust policy in place for screening to detect malnutrition because it:

- is a common and costly problem
- can adversely affect health, level of function and recovery, in both the short and long terms
- can be treated.

Without the routine use of a screening tool, there is no clear means of checking whether a patient's nutritional needs are being met and whether they are at risk of malnutrition. Other clinical assessments may not address nutritional issues. If staff do not acknowledge the importance of nutrition to a patient and its impact on their recovery from illness, the patient's nutritional state may worsen and important referrals to other healthcare professionals may be missed. Losing weight should not be considered as an inevitable part of ageing or illness. Screening is an important tool in preventing and treating malnutrition and should be an integral part of the assessment process on admission to hospital.

In order to facilitate a screening programme in your area incorporating routine screening, monitoring, assessment and treatment plans (including referral to a dietitian), the following tips may be helpful:

- Establish a clear policy locally that ensures nutrition screening is being undertaken in all clinical areas and is repeated as appropriate (NICE guidelines are a useful resource). It should include details of any areas that are exempt from routine screening, e.g. day-surgery patients. Ensure that staff at a clinical level are aware of the content of the policy and the standards they are expected to meet.
- Obtain agreement at all levels on the screening tool to be used locally, in particular that it is validated and that staff at a clinical level find it simple and quick to use (or it will not be used).
- Ensure there are appropriate resources available to provide a rolling programme of education for all staff involved in the screening process across the healthcare settings. Even after the initial education has been provided and the screening process established, education will still be required as new staff are appointed or as an update (as bad practices can set in).
- Design locally agreed care plans for monitoring and treating those patients identified as being at risk by the screening process.
- Ensure that any equipment required for the screening process is available, e.g. weighing scales, tape measure etc., is within easy access and, where appropriate, regularly calibrated. Ensure staff know where the equipment is kept and how to use it!
- Establish criteria for those requiring more detailed nutrition assessment and dietetic referral; this will vary locally, as will the resources available. This should be agreed, therefore, at a local level.

- Set up systems for the documentation of results from screening, monitoring and treatment.
- Audit the efficacy of the screening programme regularly. To ensure ownership of the process, it may be useful to encourage participation of clinical staff in the audit process.

Nutrition assessment

Nutrition assessment is a detailed, specific and in-depth appraisal of an individual's nutritional state. It should be conducted by someone with nutritional expertise, and is a fundamental component of dietetic practice. A thorough assessment of a patient's nutritional status is essential to identify the extent of malnutrition and ensure the provision of adequate and appropriate nutritional care.

Regular reassessments will also allow the success of any therapy initiated to be evaluated and plans of care to be adjusted.

There are many ways of assessing nutritional status, including:

- clinical history
- dietary history
- physical examination
- anthropometric measurements
- muscle-function tests
- biochemical data
- immunological tests.

However, the most powerful diagnostic tools are a comprehensive history and a thorough physical examination undertaken with the awareness that an inadequate nutritional status will be a problem.

Clinical history

Chronic or acute illness, injury or surgery can all have a considerable impact on a patient's nutritional status, both directly and indirectly. Dependent on the type of illness experienced, the patient could develop an increase in nutritional requirements, increased nutrient losses and/or impaired nutrient ingestion, digestion or absorption.

Medication can also affect appetite, and therefore nutrient intake, and the absorption, metabolism and excretion of nutrients, particularly in the elderly, where there may be issues of polypharmacy.

Taking a clinical history usually includes a description of the patient, relevant environmental, social and familial factors, as well as specific information regarding their medical history and that of their close family. Information regarding food allergies or intolerances should also be obtained.

This information can help establish whether a nutrient deficiency is likely to be primary, i.e. resulting from an inadequate dietary intake, or secondary in origin. A secondary deficiency may occur even when the diet is adequate. Other factors such as the medication or the patient's disease state may interfere with ingestion, absorption, transport, utilisation or excretion of the nutrient.

Clinical history is useful in the advanced stages of nutrient depletion, when overt disease is present.

Physical examination

A simple observation, or 'eyeball assessment', of an individual can provide an indication of their nutritional status (Table 3.1).

A detailed description and photographs of the physical signs of malnutrition recommended for assessment purposes by the World Health Organization (WHO) Expert Committee on Medical Assessment of Nutritional Status can be found in the *Assessment of Nutritional Status of the Community* (Jelliffe, 1966).

When assessing the patient, it is important to consider:

- **Clothing and jewellery:** Has the patient or carer noticed clothing becoming looser? Loose rings or dentures can also demonstrate weight loss.
- **Dehydration:** Does the patient have sunken eyes, a dry mouth or fragile skin? Are they confused? These can be signs of dehydration.
- **Fluid retention:** Is there any evidence of this, such as swollen ankles?
- **Mood:** Is the patient low in mood? This may affect appetite, as well as being a symptom of poor nutrition. Apathy and lethargy can be signs of malnutrition.
- **Mobility:** Has the patient's level of mobility reduced? This may be a side effect of malnutrition, and it may also compound the problem, if the individual is less able to obtain, prepare or eat food.
- **Pressure ulcers:** Poor wound healing or the presence of open wounds or ulcers will increase the patient's nutritional requirements, which if not recognised may lead to further nutritional deficiencies.

Table 3.1 Functional changes as a consequence of malnutrition

	Normal	Signs associated with malnutrition
Physical appearance	Shiny, firm hair, not easily plucked	Hair dull, dry, lack of natural shine, thin and sparse, easily plucked
	Uniform skin colour with a smooth, healthy appearance, not swollen	Swollen face, skin-colour loss, lumpiness or flakiness of skin of nose or mouth, scaling of skin around nostrils
	Shiny, clear, bright eyes	Eye membranes pale, dry, cornea has dull appearance, scar on cornea
	Lips smooth, not chapped or swollen	Redness and swelling of mouth or lips, especially at corners of mouth
	Tongue deep red in appearance, not swollen or smooth	Swelling scarlet and raw tongue, magenta colour of tongue, smooth tongue, swollen sores
	Gums healthy red, not swollen, do not bleed	Gums 'spongy' and bleed easily, recession of gums
	Nails firm and pink	Nails are spoon-shaped, brittle and ridged
Musculature	Good muscle tone, some fat under skin, can walk and run without pain	Muscles have 'wasted' appearance, bleeding into muscle (musculoskeletal haemorrhages), bow legs or knock knees, unable to get up or walk properly
Cardiovascular system	Normal heart rate and rhythm, normal blood pressure	Heart rate above 100 (tachycardia), enlarged heart, abnormal rhythm, elevated blood pressure
Nervous system	Psychological stability, normal reflexes	Mental irritability and confusion, loss of position and vibratory sense, weakness and tenderness of muscles, reduction and loss of ankle and knee reflexes, burning and tingling of hands and feet

- **Breathlessness:** This will affect the ability to eat, and possibly the ability to obtain and prepare food. It may also be a symptom of anaemia.
- **Oedema:** The presence of oedema may mask weight loss, and loss of lean muscle tissue.
- **Weight loss:** Unintentional weight loss, especially if rapid, is a concern in all patients, regardless of their original weight. Rapid weight loss tends to result in a disproportionate loss of lean muscle tissue.
- **Physical/psychosocial conditions:** Disability, social isolation or poverty can affect the ability to obtain, prepare and consume a nutritionally appropriate diet.

Dietary history

This will look at whether current nutritional needs are being met, and to what extent: current food and fluid intake, duration of any changes in appetite and intake, the presence of any other factors that may affect food and fluid intake, such as any physical or metabolic factors or whether there has been any difficulty buying, preparing or eating food.

Anthropometric measurements

Anthropometry is the external measurement of body composition, which can give important information regarding a patient's nutritional status. In 1996, the WHO published guidelines on the use of anthropometry within different population and age groups. The use of anthropometric measurement has since become accepted in clinical practice.

Commonly used anthropometric measurements include:

- body weight
- height
- adiposity (e.g. waist circumference, skinfold thickness, BMI)
- muscle mass (e.g. mid-arm muscle circumference, grip strength).

Body weight

A single measurement of body weight is of little value in assessing nutritional status, other than in order to determine BMI. It is essen-

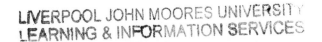

tial to obtain a regular measurement of body weight, using either the same set of scales, or calibrated scales, to determine weight changes over a period of time and to allow for an accurate calculation of the percentage of weight change. The patient should be weighed at a similar time of day on each occasion wearing similar-weight clothing, to minimise additional and inaccurate fluctuations in weight.

Quetelet's index (or BMI) is easily calculated in adults using the following formula:

$$\frac{\text{weight in kg}}{(\text{height in m})^2}$$

It is considered to be the best method of calculating BMI for most adult populations. The reason for this is that is has a low level of bias from height.

However, the categories of BMI (i.e. underweight, healthy and obese) classified by the WHO (1998) vary slightly for differing population groups, for example:

- a healthy BMI in Caucasians is 20–25, whilst in Asian, Caribbean, African and Aboriginal populations it is 18.5–23.
- an overweight BMI varies from 25 to 30 in Caucasians, 23 to 26 in Asian, Caribbean, African and Aboriginal populations and 26 to 32 in Polynesian populations.

Unfortunately, the Quetelet index does not have the ability to distinguish between excessive weight produced by adiposity, muscularity or oedema. Consequently, an extremely muscular individual may be classified as overweight or obese when, in fact, they are very lean indeed.

Percentage weight change can be calculated by:

$$\text{Weight change}\,(\%) = \frac{\text{usual weight in kg} - \text{actual weight in kg}}{\text{Usual weight in kg}} \times 100$$

Weight loss is an important indicator when assessing for malnutrition and for considering when to start nutrition support. NICE (2006) recommends considering nutrition support when:

- the patient has experienced unintentional weight loss of >10% over a three- to six-month period, or

- if the patient has a BMI of <20 kg/m^2 and has an unintentional weight loss of >5% over a three- to six-month period.

Sometimes, owing to the patient's clinical condition or a lack of suitable equipment, it is impossible to obtain an actual weight. Where these circumstances arise, it is not acceptable simply not to record a weight; instead, a surrogate weight should be obtained.

A surrogate weight can be obtained in several ways:

- From the individual: they are often aware of their weight at some point before their admission and will be able to tell you whether they have gained or lost weight recently. Bear in mind, however, that there tends to be an underestimation of weight in the obese patient and an overestimation in the underweight (Rowland, 1990; Roberts, 1995). The reported figure is also unlikely to take into account any weight change since the onset of an illness or hospital admission.
- From relatives, carers and healthcare professionals: they often offer a 'guesstimated weight'. It has been shown that first-degree relatives can often estimate weight to within 3% to 5% of measured weight (Reed & Price, 1998).
- Where it is not possible to obtain an actual or surrogate weight: other anthropometric measurements may be used, such as mid-upper-arm circumference, which has a linear relationship with weight. Such measurements would usually be undertaken by a dietitian.

It is important to recognise that a number of factors can adversely affect the accuracy of body weight measurements and should therefore be interpreted with caution:

- In the presence of oedema, ascites or fluid retention.
- The accuracy of scales used: weighing scales used in clinical areas should be of a medical grade standard and should be calibrated at least annually. Your average bathroom scales are not built for repeated use in the hospital environment.
- The time of day the patient is being weighed and the amount of clothing worn: Ideally, weights should be collected from the same set of scales, at roughly the same time of day, with the individual wearing similar clothing on each occasion.
- Amputations/false joints/splints and plaster casts can all affect the reliability and accuracy of the weight.

Height

Equipment to measure height is usually less available than weighing scales. Fortunately, most people have some idea of their height. Self-reported height is the superior measure of choice when standing height cannot be measured, even though individuals, particularly the elderly, tend to overestimate their height by up to 2 cm, as they are unaware of the reduction in height with advancing age (Rowland, 1990; Spencer *et al.*, 2002). Using an estimated height is unlikely to affect the calculation of BMI significantly. Where it is not possible to obtain a height measurement or the patient is unable to recall their height, an estimated height is a suitable alternative. Estimated height by relatives/carers has been shown to be accurate to within 1% of actual height (Reed & Price, 1998).

Muscle-function tests

Muscle-function tests assess changes in muscle contractility, relaxation rate and endurance.

These changes are thought to occur as a response to the reduction in protein stores and resulting muscle catabolism during protein-energy malnutrition.

Biochemical data

Laboratory assessments are used primarily to detect subclinical deficiency states or to confirm a clinical diagnosis. They are an objective means of assessing nutritional status, independent of emotional and other subjective factors. They are, however, often affected by factors other than those caused by depleted body stores of a nutrient, which can make an interpretation of the results difficult and confusing.

Examples of these confounding factors include:

- disease state
- level of inflammatory stress
- weight loss
- nutrient interactions
- hormonal status
- the presence of infection
- age, gender and ethnic group
- haemolysis: for serum/plasma
- recent dietary intake.

Where possible, every effort should be taken to ensure the effect of each of these factors is minimised. There should also be a standard procedure for collecting and recording samples to minimise the risk of inappropriate or inaccurate results.

Some biochemical tests monitor short-term or acute changes in nutritional status; others provide a longer-term picture of nutritional status. Providing details of all the biochemical tests available is beyond the scope of this book, but further reading can be found in *Essentials of Human Nutrition* (Mann & Truswell, 2005).

Immunologic function tests

Immunocompetence can be assessed by the delayed cutaneous hyper-sensitivity (DCH) response. Specific antigens are injected intradermally into the forearm, and the induced response is noted. In healthy individuals, T-cells respond by proliferation and the release of soluble mediators of inflammation, resulting in redness and hardening at the site. In malnourished individuals, with protein-energy malnutrition and/or nutrient deficiencies (such as zinc, iron and vitamin A), these reactions are often reduced, but can be reversed with nutritional rehabilitation.

It is worth noting that many non-nutritional factors can make interpreting the immunological tests more complicated.

Screening tools

For nutrition screening to be effective, it is important to use a screening tool that is:

- Practical
  - Quick and easy to use and understand
  - Has a range of alternative measures when height and weight cannot be measured
- Universal
  - Can be used in adults of all ages, regardless of state of health
  - Is applicable across different care settings (hospital, GP practice, nursing home, free living)
  - Allows continuity of care
  - Can be used for public health purposes

- Reliable
  - ○ Good reproducibility between users
  - ○ Good internal reliability
- Evidence-based and peer-reviewed
- Linked to a care plan for treatment
  - ○ Facilitates nursing and other staff initiating appropriate monitoring or treatment and referral to the dietitian or Nutrition Support Team
- Developed by a multidisciplinary group for use by all healthcare professionals
- Acceptable to patients and healthcare professionals
- Has a method of scoring in place that clearly identifies patients who are:
  - ○ Low risk: no immediate action; repeat screening at regular intervals to detect any change
  - ○ Moderate risk: need ongoing monitoring to detect any change
  - ○ High risk: require intervention and ongoing monitoring

(Nursing and Midwifery Practice Development Unit, 2002; Stratton, 2007)

There are many screening tools available. Indeed, Green and Watson (2005) identify 71 nutrition screening/assessment tools used by nurses, many of which they highlight as not having been subjected to rigorous testing. The use of differing tools between organisations makes it difficult to transfer results from one area to another. The MUST (Malnutrition Universal Screening Tool) is one that fulfils the criteria required for a successful screening tool. MUST is supported by the British Dietetic Association, the Royal College of Nursing, the Royal College of Physicians (England) and the Registered Nursing Homes Association. In Scotland, nutrition screening of hospital patients is mandatory and the tool suggested for use is MUST (NHS Quality Improvement Scotland, 2003). MUST is also recommended by the 2006 NICE guidance *Nutrition Support in Adults*.

MUST was developed by the Malnutrition Advisory Group of BAPEN, and can be applied to all types of patient groups (Stratton *et al.*, 2004). It has been designed to identify those at risk of malnutrition, together with those who are obese. It has not been designed to detect poor vitamin and mineral status (Stratton, 2007).

MUST has been developed for use in:

- all adults
- hospital wards

- out-patient clinics
- general practice
- community settings.

Documentation

All nutrition screening documentation should be kept, and reviewed, and repeated where appropriate on a weekly basis. The initial screen acts as a baseline against which to monitor progress and the achievement of targets. Without a baseline screening result and/or assessment, it becomes very difficult to determine the efficacy and cost-effectiveness of any treatment instigated. It also acts as evidence that nutrition screening has been conducted, and shows which nutritional care plan was implemented.

All equipment required to complete assessments should be accessible and in good working order. It should be maintained and calibrated regularly, and documentation that this has been conducted should be available. This should be done as a minimum standard on an annual basis.

When to refer to a dietitian

Although there may be small differences in referral criteria at a local level, most Trusts have a policy and procedure for referral to a dietitian. There may be differences in who is able to make the referral, but ultimately reasons for referral will be similar. Often referral will be where there is a high nutritional risk score, indicating a high risk of malnutrition, where nutrition support is required or whether there is the need for a more detailed dietary assessment.

Following screening, nursing staff will often have started recording food and fluid intake and may have introduced dietary supplements. The next step would be to refer on to the dietitian if there has been no improvement in nutritional intake. It is usually of benefit to the dietitian to specify a level of urgency, as sometimes routine referrals will not be seen for several days, depending on staffing levels, caseload and whether a dietetic department is on site.

To avoid delaying treatment, when referring a patient nursing staff should provide the dietitian with the following information:

- the patient's weight
- their nutritional risk score

- a valid reason for referral
- evidence that the nursing actions, often documented on the screening tool, have been undertaken (e.g. intake charts, starting a high-protein diet).

The patient should be referred:

- if the screening tool highlights any risk of malnutrition
- if their nutritional state does not improve even when nursing actions have been completed
- for further assessment
- where nutrition support is required
- according to local policy and criteria.

Conclusion

A continued commitment to nutrition screening at a clinical level can be an effective driver in identifying patients who are malnourished, ensuring referrals are made to the other healthcare professionals, starting appropriate nutritional care and raising the importance of nutrition for patients in hospital.

References

Allison, S.P. (1999) *Hospital Food as Treatment: A report by a working party of the British Association for Parenteral and Enteral Nutrition*, BAPEN, Maidenhead.

British Association for Parenteral and Enteral Nutrition (2007) National Screening Week (NSW), http://www.bapen.org.uk/res_press_rel37.html, accessed 12 January 2008.

Department of Health (2001) *National Service Framework for Older People*, DH, London.

Green, S.M., Watson, R. (2005) Nutritional screening and assessment tools for use by nurses: Literature review. *Journal of Advanced Nursing* **50** (1), 69–83.

Jelliffe, D.B. (1966) *The Assessment of the Nutritional Status of the Community*, WHO Monograph Series No. 53, World Health Organization, Geneva.

Mann, J., Truswell, S.A. (2005) *Essentials of Human Nutrition*, 3rd edn, Oxford University Press, New York.

National Institute for Health and Clinical Excellence (2006) *Nutrition Support in Adults: Oral nutrition support, enteral tube feeding and parenteral nutrition, Clinical Guideline 32*, NICE, London.

NHS Quality Improvement Scotland (2003) *Standard for Hospital Food, Fluid and Nutritional Care in Hospitals*, NHS QIS, Edinburgh.

Nursing and Midwifery Practice Development Unit (2002) *Nutrition Assessment and Referral for Adults in Hospital Best Practice Statement*, NMPDU, NHS Scotland, Edinburgh.

Reed, D.R., Price, R.A. (1998) Estimates of the heights and weights of family members: Accuracy of informant reports. *International Journal of Obesity* **22** (9), 827–35.

Roberts, R.J. (1995) Can self-reported data accurately describe the prevalence of overweight? *Public Health* **109** (4), 275–84.

Rowland, M.L. (1990) Self-reported weight and height. *American Journal of Clinical Nutrition* **52**, 1125–33.

Spencer, E.A., Appleby, P.N., Davey, G.K., Key, T.J. (2002) Validity of self-reported height and weight in 4808 EPIC-Oxford participants. *Public Health Nutrition* **5** (4), 561–5.

Stratton, R. (2007) Malnutrition (Chapter 1.10), in *Manual of Dietetic Practice*, 4th edn (eds B. Thomas and J. Bishop), Blackwell Publishing, Oxford.

Stratton, R.J., King, C.L., Stroud, M.A. *et al.* (2004) 'Malnutrition Universal Screening Tool' predicts mortality and length of hospital stay in acutely ill elderly. *British Journal of Nutrition* **95**, 325–30.

World Health Organization (1996) Anthropometric reference data for international use: Recommendations from a WHO Expert Committee. American Journal of Clinical Nutrition **64**, 650–8.

World Health Organization (1998) *Obesity: Preventing and Managing the Global Epidemic. Report of a WHO Consultation on Obesity*, Geneva, 3–5 June 1997, WHO, Geneva.

Further reading

Department of Health (2007) *Improving Nutritional Care: A Joint Action Plan from the Department of Health and Nutrition Summit Stakeholders*, DH, London.

Chapter 4

The Nursing Role in Maintaining Patients' Oral Nutritional Intake

Carolyn Best

Introduction

Nutrition plays a vital role in the patient's recovery process and, whilst it could be argued that nutrition is everyone's responsibility, registered nurses have traditionally played a central role in meeting the nutritional needs of patients in hospital.

The extent of nurses' involvement in the nutritional care of patients has varied over time, reflecting the changing perceptions of the public and of nurses themselves about the nature of their responsibilities. In the late nineteenth and early twentieth centuries, a hospital matron was the active head of the nursing staff and had charge of the kitchen and nursing arrangements.

During the mid-twentieth century, this role was changed as matrons and senior nurses relinquished direct managerial control of catering and housekeeping functions making it increasingly difficult to influence the standards of care provided by these groups of staff (Royal College of Nursing, 2005). Towards the end of the twentieth century, the contracting-out of catering services has made the process even more difficult. In addition, as nursing roles have expanded, the level of importance attributed to patient nutrition at ward level has diminished and responsibilities have become blurred. This lack of engagement is highlighted in a report by the Association of Community Health Councils for England and Wales (1997), which suggests that some nurses were withdrawing totally from facilitating the delivery of meals and providing patients with the appropriate assistance required to eat.

Two reports published by the Royal College of Nursing (RCN), *Nutritional Standards and the Older Adult* (1993) and *Statement on Feeding and Nutrition in Hospitals* (1996), identify the responsibilities of the nurse in relation to patient nutrition, but unfortunately neither clarifies the responsibility of the registered nurse in providing physical assistance to aid patients with their meals. In an attempt to remedy the situation, the UK Central Council for Nursing, Midwifery and Health Visiting (UKCC) published a registrar's letter (1997) stating the role of the registered nurse in feeding patients:

> Nurses have a responsibility to report to an appropriate person or authority and circumstances in which safe and appropriate care for patients or clients cannot be provided . . . While registered nurses may of course delegate the tasks of feeding patients, for example to unregistered practitioners, the overall responsibility lies with the registered nurse.

It appeared to have little impact, as a report released by the Department of Health in 1999, *Not Because They Are Old*, provides evidence that nurses were not recognising or responding to patients who had difficulty eating their food.

Policy introduced at the beginning of this century has led to national initiatives aimed at improving nutritional care for patients in hospital, including the *Essence of Care Toolkit* (Department of Health, 2001a) and the *Better Hospital Food Programme* (NHS Estates, 2001a), but despite these initiatives problems with patient nutrition are still a regular occurrence (Age Concern, 2006).

Identifying the problems

The standard of nutritional care delivered to patients is reliant upon a number of factors, including:

- the level of nutritional knowledge and organisational skills of registered nurses in the clinical area.
- their involvement at patient meals; the many reasons cited for why nurses do not become involved in patient nutrition include:
  - nurses consider nutrition and feeding as basic care
  - patient nutrition is delegated to student nurses and domestic staff
  - nurses may have negative attitudes to nutrition and feeding, particularly with older people, who are sometimes difficult to feed, underweight or seen as messy eaters
  - it takes too much time
  - poor nutritional knowledge

    o   a lack of understanding of the importance of nutrition
    o   changes in the way meals are delivered to wards.
        (Carr & Mitchell, 1991; British Association for Parenteral and
        Enteral Nutrition, 1999; Council of Europe, 2002)

- the skills and knowledge of healthcare assistants supporting registered nurses:
  If nurses delegate the responsibility for meal distribution and providing patient assistance, they are less likely to be aware of their patients' nutritional intake or any eating/swallowing problems. Without training, unqualified staff may not have the knowledge or skill to assist patients who have chewing/swallowing difficulties or to help them make an informed choice in selecting an appropriate meal from the menu.

- poor communication between nursing staff, healthcare assistants, catering and domestic/housekeeping staff.
  There needs to be a clear two-way communication channel where each group of staff is aware of its responsibilities and the level of information that it is required to feedback (Table 4.1). Often there is a culture of blame where the only communication between clinical areas and the catering department is when problems arise. In this situation, it becomes relatively easy to focus on the negative side of hospital food and catering – to the detriment of the patient and their nutritional intake.

Registered nurse responsibilities in patient nutrition

Leadership

Nurses have a key role to play in the promotion and maintenance of good nutritional care through the clear management of patient mealtimes and through enhancing the mealtime environment, for example protected mealtimes. Where there is a lack of leadership or ownership, mistakes can be made, leading to an increased risk of patients receiving incorrect or inadequate dietary requirements. Delays in serving food or incorrectly delivered meals will not encourage the patient to eat the food they are provided or to view hospital food in a positive light. Identifying one person to coordinate the serving of meals should help to ensure that those patients who need assistance to eat their meal receive the appropriate level of help they require.

Carr and Mitchell (1991) demonstrate that qualified nurses are more likely to be involved with mealtimes when they are expected to serve

Table 4.1 Roles and responsibilities

Role	Responsibilities	Reports to	Actions required/Information reported
Nursing staff	Ensuring the patient receives appropriate nutrition	1. Care assistants	1a. Specific patient care required at mealtimes 1b. Ensuring all staff are aware of the patient's dietary and fluid requirements
		2. Catering department	2a. Ordering appropriate patient meals using menus 2b. Feeding back problems/advising that alternative meals are required 2c. Additional meals required
		3. Domestic/housekeeping staff	3a. Patients with fluid restrictions 3b. Patients who will require longer periods to eat their meals 3c. Feedback that is required when food trays are cleared on completion of a meal
Care assistants	Under the direction of the qualified nurse, ensuring the patient receives appropriate nutrition	1. Nursing staff	1a. Amount of food eaten by patients 1b. Level of assistance required to eat/drink 1c. Problems with swallowing 1d. Record food and fluid intake on completion of a meal or snack
		2. Catering department	2. Support the role of the qualified nurse
		3. Domestic/housekeeping staff	3. Support the role of the qualified nurse
Catering department	Provide appropriate meals that are nutritionally balanced as agreed by the menus distributed	1. Nursing staff	1a. To provide appropriate meals/specialist diets according to ward requests via menus 1b. To feedback to ward areas when problems arise in providing the meals/diets requested
Domestic/housekeeping staff	• Keep the patient's environment clean • Provide water and hot drinks for the patient • Clear away food trays on completion of a meal	1. Nursing staff	1a. Check if patients are nil by mouth or fluid restricted before delivering water jugs to the bedside 1b. Feedback those patients who have not eaten meals or problems that were reported when food trays collected

meals onto plates and deliver those meals to patients. Where meals arrive on the ward already plated and placed on individually named trays, the involvement of qualified nurses is minimal.

Coordination of mealtimes should extend to ensuring that all food and fluid charts are completed when a meal or snack has been eaten and any identified problems are reported back to the coordinator/qualified nurse.

On a more strategic level, to highlight issues affecting nutritional care at a clinical level, nurses should work closely with catering, dietetic and domestic staff to develop systems and procedures which will support the complex issue of food and drink provision within hospital.

Nutrition screening

Nutrition screening is clearly part of the nurse's role. Nurses are in the ideal position and have the appropriate skills to enable them to accurately screen the patient on admission (or soon afterwards) to identify those at risk of malnutrition and to assess their nutritional needs. The National Institute for Health and Clinical Excellence (2006) states that all hospital patients should be screened on admission and the screening process should be repeated weekly where there is clinical concern.

Appropriate referral for those with complex nutritional needs

To ensure that appropriate nutritional care is provided, it is essential that on completion of nutrition screening nurses follow and implement the appropriate care guidelines that accompany the screening tool. Nurses often do not recognise the important role they play in providing nutritional care to the patient and it is not uncommon for the nutrition screening tool to have been completed and the patient referred to a dietitian before the nursing actions recommended on the screening tool have been implemented. In some patients, if the nursing actions are followed, it may not be necessary to refer the patient to the dietitian.

Nursing actions listed on a screening tool may include:

- the completion of a food chart for three days
- the use of a fortified drink or pudding to supplement a patient's dietary intake, as in the case of the elderly patient who cannot manage to eat enough of a normal diet
- recording regular weights.

Conversely, it is also important for nurses to recognise when the patient has complex nutritional needs and when immediate referral to a dietitian is essential.

Ensuring patients eat the food provided

Neither a nutrition screening process nor a dietetic nutrition assessment will be of benefit to the patient unless the results are acted upon and the patient eats the food provided to them. It is the responsibility of the nurse caring for the patient to ensure that they receive their food and that they are provided with the appropriate level of encouragement or assistance to enable them to eat.

There are a number of measures that, if implemented, will help to increase the amount of food the patient is likely to eat at mealtimes:

- Select meals as close to mealtimes as possible.
- Provide patients with the opportunity to select meals from menu cards that they can read and understand and that where necessary assistance is provided to choose meals.
- Clearly record patients' food preferences, their dietary requirements and their ability to manage food and fluids.
- Provide, where appropriate, access to fresh drinking water.
- Assess and clearly record what level of assistance is required for feeding.
- Ensure staff are available during mealtimes to ensure that the appropriate level of assistance is provided to patients.

Education to deliver and monitor appropriate nutritional care

All nurses involved in the clinical care of patients should receive education both pre- and post registration regarding the importance of good nutrition, the implications of malnutrition, nutrition screening and techniques for providing nutrition support. Education should provide nurses with the knowledge to make appropriate assessments and/or referrals, identify individual patient's nutritional needs and highlight ways of improving patients' nutritional intake.

If nurses can appreciate the important role nutrition plays in the patient's recovery from illness, attitudes and standards of nutritional care provided will improve.

Programmes should be tailored to the needs of the clinical area and to the level at which the staff attending are practising.

Documentation

Documentation should include a clear and visible account of the:

- patient's height and weight
- their nutrition screening tool score
- any involuntary or unintentional weight loss (over the previous three months), including visual indicators such as loose clothing, rings or dentures
- nursing actions taken on completion of the screening tool
- nutrition care plans
- patient allergies
- their food preferences
- any relevant medical condition
- medication that may affect patient's appetite
- dietary and fluid intake
- special diets required
- patient's appetite status, e.g. appetite nil or virtually nil
- patient's ability to take food orally
- level of assistance required to eat
- presence of severe vomiting and/or diarrhoea.

Discharge documentation should incorporate details of the patient's nutritional status, any special dietary or equipment requirements and any community/out-patient follow-up required.

Dysphagia screening

Dysphagia-trained nurses are educated to:

- screen for signs of oropharyngeal dysphagia
- assess and manage simple oral swallowing problems
- recognise swallowing problems that may arise during feeding
- follow safe swallowing recommendations
- prepare and monitor a range of consistencies and textures
- select appropriate utensils/containers
- feed patients without putting them at risk of aspirating
- know when to refer to a speech and language therapist for further assessment.

A dysphagia-trained nurse will normally undertake the first swallow assessment at ward level for patients they suspect to be at risk of dysphagia, before referring the patient to a speech and

Box 4.1 Role of the HCA at mealtimes

1. Assist patients to complete menus.
2. Assist the patient to sit appropriately in preparation for a meal.
3. Give patients the opportunity to wash their hands.
4. Ensure dentures are fitted and the oral cavity is clean.
5. Deliver the correct meal to the correct patient.
6. Place food within patient's reach.
7. Open tops and cut up food.
8. Provide verbal encouragement to eat.
9. Provide supplements/helping patient to drink.
10. Complete food and fluid charts.
11. Record weight.
12. Provide physical assistance to eat.
13. Report any patient difficulties or lack of nutritional intake back to the registered nurse.

language therapist. This role is particularly helpful in minimising delays in commencing nutritional intake (oral or artificial enteral) if patient assessment is required outside the hours that speech and language therapists are available.

The responsibilities of the healthcare assistant

The healthcare assistant (HCA) has an equally important role to play in ensuring patients receive their nutritional requirements (Box 4.1). In reality, it is often the HCA who takes the lead in completing patient menus and distributing meals in clinical areas. It is therefore in the interest of the patient, nurse and HCA to ensure they are equipped with the appropriate level of skill and knowledge to provide patients with the help and support they need.

Roles and responsibilities of other individuals involved in patient nutrition

Relatives/volunteers

Relatives, carers or a trained volunteer can play a very important role in assisting patients in hospital to eat or drink at mealtimes. Some patients may feel uncomfortable eating amongst strangers, particularly if they have a disability making eating difficult, experi-

Box 4.2   Issues to be reported to nursing staff

1. If the patient has a problem initiating a swallow.
2. Sudden coughing during or immediately after swallowing.
3. Food remaining in the mouth after swallowing.
4. A wet or gurgly voice after swallowing.
5. Excess dribbling of saliva, food or fluid from lips.
6. Long delays in chewing food and moving it to the back of the mouth.
7. Patient becomes drowsy.

ence dysphagia or only manage to eat very slowly. The offer of assistance from someone not in uniform may make them feel more comfortable and encourage them to eat more of their meal than they would have done if left to manage independently. Assistance provided by ward staff makes some patients feel they need to rush their meal as they feel they are taking the nurse away from other important responsibilities. Assistance from a relative or volunteer may make the patient feel more comfortable about eating, and so make them feel more in control and so more likely to increase their nutritional intake.

For some patients, packaged foods may prove difficult to open. They may feel reluctant to ask for help. A relative or volunteer is ideally placed to help open packages, cut up meat, position cutlery or crockery or put straws in cartons. These simple but essential actions may be all that is required to maintain the patient's independence.

When using relatives or volunteers to support patients at mealtimes, it is essential that they are:

- clear on how best to provide assistance safely to the patient
- clear of the boundaries of their role
- aware of the reporting structure for problems or concerns
- aware of the information that should be reported (Box 4.2)
- made aware of any feeding or fluid restrictions or special dietary requirements

Ward housekeepers

In 2001, the Department of Health recommended that NHS Trusts appoint ward housekeepers to maximise the effectiveness of the modern matrons (Department of Health, 2001b) and that 50% of hospitals should have ward housekeepers in post by the end of 2004.

The responsibilities of the housekeeper may include some or all of the following tasks:

- cleaning
- ensuring meals meet patients' needs
- helping patients complete menu cards
- chasing up special diets
- providing assistance for patients who require feeding
- improving communication between facilities and clinical staff

Management of the role of housekeeper differs across organisations with some being responsible to domestic or catering departments, but it was intended by NHS Estates (2001b) that ward housekeepers should work within the ward team and be responsible to the ward sister/manager.

Link nurses

Link nurses are part of a system that disseminates appropriate, relevant information in a specialist area and provides a route for formal, two-way communication between their colleagues in the clinical area and the specialist team they represent, for example nutrition, infection control and tissue viability.

A successful link nurse system depends upon:

- the effectiveness of the link nurses to act as role models and to disseminate information to their clinical colleagues
- a recognition of their extended role in the workplace
- their ability to influence practice on their wards and beyond
- the feedback of information to specialist teams to direct education sessions and influence future practice.

When used appropriately, link nurses should gain an increased awareness of the specialist area they represent and how it affects the patient's pathway. The appropriate use of this system has the potential to promote and enhance clinical effectiveness and disseminate research findings.

However, for this system to work effectively the link nurse has to commit to the role. They must recognise that they are attending meetings not just to update their own knowledge and skills but also to share them amongst their clinical colleagues to improve their practice. Some protected time is advantageous to develop the role, but ongoing support and encouragement from ward teams and clinical managers is essential to maintain the role. Without this, a valuable resource could be lost.

The patient in hospital

As the patient arrives in a hospital ward, they are introduced into a situation and setting over which they often have little or no control. They relinquish their day-to-day responsibilities and are forced to adopt a more passive role. Often, one of the first actions required of the patient is to change into their nightwear; even if they do not feel unwell on admission to the ward, they will almost certainly need to have a surgical gown on for when investigations are undertaken or treatment is begun.

In our experience, there are a number of reasons why a patient's nutritional intake reduces in hospital (Box 4.3), and it is therefore not surprising that during this time many patients lose weight.

These issues do little to promote the improvement or maintenance of a person's dietary intake. Finding solutions to these varied

---

Box 4.3 Patients' reasons for not eating in hospital

1. Hospital mealtimes are too inflexible: would eat earlier or later at home or would have main meal in the evening not the middle of the day.
2. Do not like the taste, smell or appearance of food.
3. Problems in ordering food: some people may require help in menu completion because of poor comprehension, language difficulties, poor sight, an inability to physically complete the menu or illiteracy.
4. The meal delivered is not the meal the patient ordered.
5. The type or consistency of diet delivered is incorrect.
6. Feeling unwell.
7. Lack of appropriate utensils.
8. Food tray placed out of reach.
9. Lack of availability of staff to assist patients to eat.
10. Mealtimes are disrupted by ward rounds, investigations or procedures.
11. Restrictions on the amount of time a patient has to eat a meal before it is removed.
12. Patient absent from the ward when meals are delivered.
13. Being placed nil by mouth (NBM) whilst awaiting swallow assessment.
14. A breakdown in communication between nursing, catering and/or dietetic staff.

problems is not necessarily costly, in terms of finances, but does depend upon the availability (and commitment) of specialist staff (Department of Health, 1999).

Recommendations to improve patient intake

1. Nutritionally screen patients to highlight level of nutritional risk.
   Follow the nursing action plan detailed on the screening tool to provide the appropriate level of nutritional care required. Refer the patient to the relevant healthcare professional as appropriate (e.g. speech therapist, dietitian).
2. Provide assistance with menu choice/completion.
   Menu cards are usually sent to clinical areas on a daily basis. They set out the food choices available to patients each day, including options for special diets or food cooked to meet cultural or religious needs.
   Most patients will be able to complete their own menu card but for others it may highlight a problem. Patients with poor eyesight or difficulty reading or writing may need tactful assistance. For some groups of patients, meal names may require explanation. Although providing assistance may prove time-consuming, it is in the patient's interest to involve them in making their menu choices. Patients who are not given a menu or the opportunity to select their own meals may regard the food supplied less favourably and be unwilling or unable to eat it.
3. Place food within reach of the patient.
4. Avoid staff breaks during mealtimes and minimise disturbances to the patient mealtime, i.e. protected mealtimes.
5. Have a clearly identified leader or coordinator at mealtimes to organise the delivery of meals to patients and ensure that those patients who require assistance to eat are provided with appropriate help or utensils.
6. Determine the reasons for a patient's poor nutritional intake (Box 4.3).
   Delivering food to the patient's bedside does not guarantee that the food will be eaten. There may be a number of medical or mechanical reasons why a patient will experience difficulty in eating their meals independently, including:
   - **Psychological status**
     o   acute/chronic confusion or memory loss
     o   poor motivation to eat

- o   inability to recognise food
- o   giving the patient food that makes them different from others, e.g. puree or soft diet
- **Physical ability**
  - o   poor eyesight
  - o   appropriate assistance with meals is not provided
- **Mechanical problems**
  - o   poorly fitting or absent dentures
  - o   arthritis
- **Medical condition**
  - o   poor swallowing technique (dysphagia)
  - o   pain and discomfort
  - o   medication side effects (poor appetite, constipation, drowsiness)
  - o   nausea
  - o   NBM

7. Assess the level of assistance required.
    Nursing staff should know how best to assist a patient with their meal without taking over or undermining the patient's ability or confidence. Where the patient needs assistance to eat and drink, the nurse should provide support in a manner that encourages the patient, where appropriate, to promote or maintain independence.
    Some patients may require assistance to prepare for eating, e.g. removing food and utensils from packaging, straws pushed into cartons, bread buttered and meat cut up. Others may manage to eat independently earlier in the day or manage a first course unaided but need assistance following this. Undertaking a patient assessment will help to identify the level of assistance required.

8. Review timings of supplements.
    Giving supplements within an hour of a mealtime may result in the patient feeling too full to cope with eating a full meal. As supplements are normally prescribed to help increase nutritional intake, this action will only be to the patient's detriment. They may be best offered between meals.

9. Adverse effects of medication.
    Some elderly patients are prescribed a large number of differing medications. These medications can have a variety of side effects that can potentially influence a patient's nutritional intake. For example, medication can cause the following:
    - nausea and vomiting, e.g. opiates
    - constipation (patient can experience 'fullness'), e.g. ondanstron, opiates

- dry mouth (lack of saliva to eat food with), e.g. tricyclic antidepressants
- weight gain, e.g. oral contraceptive pill, steroids
- increased appetite, e.g. antipsychotic medications
- anorexia, e.g. drugs used in Parkinsonism
- diarrhoea (resulting in nutrition not adequately absorbed from gastrointestinal tract), e.g. magnesium supplements, artificial sweeteners)
- malabsorption of vitamins, e.g. oral liquid paraffin can reduce the absorption of vitamin A and other fat-soluble vitamins
- gastric irritation, e.g. non-steroidal anti-inflammatory drugs (Aronson, 2006)

10. Address symptoms that may affect nutritional intake, e.g. pain, nausea, dyspnoea, constipation.
11. Check that if the patient wears dentures they are cleaned, fit properly and are used!
12. Ensure the patient is positioned comfortably in as upright a position as possible (an angle of at least 30° is advisable)
13. Consider the use of an appetite stimulant where appropriate, e.g. a small glass of wine or sherry before a meal.
14. Ensure staff are aware of the process of obtaining food outside of mealtimes. Following the Better Hospital Food initiative (NHS Estates, 2001) hospitals will have some, if not all, of the following 24-hour catering provisions in place:
    - light-bite hot meals, including dishes such as cottage pie
    - light refreshments available in the ward kitchen, including tea, coffee, biscuits or fresh fruit
    - snack boxes providing sandwiches or cheese and crackers, fruit, yoghurt and a drink
15. Where oral intake is expected to be suboptimal or impossible over an extended period, consider alternative methods of providing nutrition, e.g. feeding via an enteral tube.

Safety considerations when assisting a patient to eat

Assisting a patient to eat is not without risk. The individual providing support should consider the following before placing food or fluid in the patient's mouth:

- Make sure the patient is alert and responsive and is positioned in an upright position (where possible).

- Check that the patient is not NBM.
- Communicate with the patient, maintaining eye contact to ensure you are providing food at an appropriate rate, the food is not too hot or too cold and that the patient has eaten enough. Limit interruptions and distractions.
- Check the patient is receiving the correct diet, e.g. whether they require a high-protein diet, soft/purée diet or low-potassium diet.
- Does the patient require thickened fluids? What consistency is required? Be aware that thickening tea, coffee or water may alter the taste.
- Pour thickened fluids into cups. Don't use a straw.
- If the patient has a purée or soft meal, let them know what they are eating, particularly if it has been ordered for them by someone else. (One purée or minced meal may look and taste similar to another.)
- Wait for the patient to finish chewing before introducing the next mouthful.
- Give small amounts of food at a time.
- Pause between mouthfuls to ensure that the patient is ready.
- Use a spoon not a fork to deliver food.
- Monitor the patient for fatigue.
- Offer meals in the usual order but be prepared that some patients find the smell of hot food nauseating and prefer the drink and dessert.
- On completion of a meal:
    o   leave the patient in an upright position
    o   complete food intake charts
    o   report and record difficulties with food consistency.

Helping the dysphagic patient to eat

Dysphagia is characterised by:

- difficulty in chewing and swallowing foods and/or liquids
- coughing or choking when eating
- food sticking in the throat or chest
- difficulty swallowing saliva.

For the patient with dysphagia, there is an increased risk of aspiration of food or liquids into the respiratory tract. It can also make taking in enough fluid and nutrients a challenge. If the problem remains untreated, the patient may develop dehydration, a declining nutritional intake and, if aspiration is present, pneumonia.

Symptoms of dysphagia may include:

- pocketing food in the cheek
- extra effort needed to chew or swallow food or fluid
- inability to swallow
- drooling
- choking or coughing while eating or immediately after meal
- wet or gurgled voice
- sensation of food sticking in throat
- bringing food or stomach acid back up (regurgitation).

If the patient aspirates during feeding, signs and symptoms may include:

- coughing
- increased sputum production
- shortness of breath.

To minimise the risk of aspiration, it may be necessary to encourage the patient to take repeated swallows and clear their throat gently after every few mouthfuls. This ensures any food residue is cleared from the throat. Modify the consistency of the patient's diet to make it easier to chew or swallow, i.e. providing a soft or purée diet.

This may be sufficient for some patients but for those with continuing severe dysphagia it may be necessary to consider alternative methods of providing nutrition, e.g. via an enteral feeding tube, depending upon their medical condition and prognosis.

Effects of dementia on oral nutritional intake

Patients with advanced dementia develop swallowing problems and an indifference to food (Hurley & Volicer, 2002), leading to risk of aspiration, reduced nutritional intake and weight loss. During mealtimes, they may exhibit a number of problems, including:

- poor appetite
- refusing to open their mouth
- holding food in their mouth or spitting food out
- turning their head away from food
- forgetting how to eat or drink
- forgetting how to use cutlery

- developing swallowing problems
- resisting the person who is trying to feed them
- throwing their food about
- comfort eating
- becoming easily distracted
- forgetting when they last ate
- eating more slowly or quickly than previously
- developing a change in taste preferences, e.g. mixing puddings in with a main meal (whilst this may be off-putting to watch, it may increase the amount the patient eats)
- becoming suspicious about food: may express panic as food gets closer to the mouth or fear of being poisoned
- jaw clamping.

As a result, these changes in eating behaviour may lead to:

- malnutrition
- weight loss
- weight gain
- dehydration
- constipation.

To maximise nutritional intake, it is important that meals should be as relaxed and unhurried as possible. Distractions should be kept to a minimum as it can prove difficult for a patient to resume eating once their focus on the meal has been broken. Some patients may eat more if they are given finger foods as they don't need to remain seated as they eat. It will also allow them to maintain their independence during eating over a longer period.

To involve the patient in the process of eating, encourage them to hold their spoon and guide it to their mouth. Avoid giving a mixture of liquid and solid as it may lead them to swallow instead of chew and could result in choking. Sometimes, a person with dementia will feel compelled to search out and consume any type of food. Apart from the problems associated with overeating, this type of behaviour can cause the person to eat or drink unsuitable, or even dangerous, substances.

Other helpful tips include:

- Remove any items from the table that may distract eating.
- Talk about the food to be eaten.
- Avoid a plateful of blandly coloured foods.
- Place drinks in coloured containers.
- Allow plenty of time between mouthfuls.

During the later stages of dementia, some people develop a taste for specific foods, and particularly foods with strong flavours. Fluids may need to be thickened to reduce the risk of aspiration.

For more information on this subject, readers should consult Department of Health (2007) or visit the Alzheimer's Society's website at www.alzheimers.org.uk.

Red trays

The 'red tray' initiative (Bradley & Rees, 2003) is a simple but effective idea that clearly indicates to staff serving meals in ward areas which patients require assistance to eat and drink.

Following the completion of a nutrition assessment, the patient's need for assistance with nutritional intake should be identified and recorded.

When meals are ordered, a clear indication is made upon the patient's menu sheet either with, for example, a red dot or 'RED TRAY' written clearly in red pen indicating to the catering department that the meal ordered for this particular patient must be placed upon a red tray. This enables the staff responsible for serving meals within a ward to instantly see how many patients require assistance at that mealtime and plan the delivery of meals appropriately. All non-red trays should be served first to patients who can manage their meals independently. This ensures that all red trays remain in the food trolley until all other trays have been delivered. Nursing staff can then offer the appropriate level of support to more needy patients. Leaving the tray in the trolley until assistance can be provided ensures the patient receives a warm meal, which they will be more likely to eat!

On completion of a meal, the red tray should not be removed by housekeeping staff until the nurse responsible for that patient's care accurately records their nutritional intake on a food chart.

For this initiative to work effectively, there needs to be clear communication between nursing staff and housekeeping staff, the catering department and temporary nursing staff.

Protected mealtimes

'Protected mealtimes' were introduced in 2004 in an attempt to minimise the amount of non-essential activity undertaken in wards during mealtimes to allow nurses to concentrate on helping patients to eat and to provide a quieter ward environment that would be more conducive to eating.

The Protected Mealtimes Campaign was launched by the Hospital Caterers Association (2004) as part of the Better Hospital Food programme with the aim of:

- providing meals that are free of avoidable and unnecessary interruptions
- creating a quiet and relaxed atmosphere in which patients are afforded time to enjoy meals
- recognising and supporting the social aspects of eating
- providing an environment that is welcoming, clean, tidy and conducive to eating
- limiting ward-based activities, including clinical tasks such as drug rounds or non-clinical tasks such as cleaning, to those that are essential or relevant to mealtimes
- focusing ward activities on the service of food so that patients are supported appropriately at mealtimes
- emphasising to all staff, patients and visitors the importance of mealtimes as part of the patient's care and treatment.

Often, one of the first actions undertaken when trying to introduce protected mealtimes is the displaying of posters at the entrance to a clinical area with the aim of informing healthcare professionals and visitors of the purpose and timing of the protected mealtime.

Whilst the use of posters plays a vital part in the implementation of this initiative, it is not the only action required. Work needs to be undertaken across whole organisations to gain the support of all healthcare professionals from board level down.

It requires the following:

- The support and knowledge of all healthcare professionals to mange their workload in a way that minimises interruptions to patients. This may mean that the order in which meal trolleys are delivered to ward areas is made common knowledge so that visits to individual wards can be planned.
- The support of the catering department as meals may be required for nursing staff outside of the traditional mealtime period. The availability of food at other times will place less pressure on nursing staff to take their meals at the same time as the meal trolley is delivered to the ward.

- Visiting times may need to be reviewed to minimise interruptions from visitors unless they are actively involved in assisting the patient to eat.

Recording food intake

For patients who are malnourished or have difficulty taking adequate amounts of food and drink, accurate completion of food and fluid charts after a meal is extremely important. However, it is not uncommon to see a poorly completed chart giving little useful information (Figure 4.1). If the patient's nutritional intake is to be accurately calculated measurable amounts of food and fluid consumed need to be obtained (Figure 4.2). Directly after a meal, the food chart should be completed by the practitioner who has assisted the patient with their meal. They should record the amount of food that the patient has eaten rather than the amount of food that was originally offered.

Day 1

Patient details: John Smith		Ward: B5
Time	**Food/Drink**	**Quantity**
Early morning	Cup of tea	200 ml
Breakfast	Cereal Orange juice	?
Mid-morning	Fortijuice	Sips
Lunchtime	Cottage pie Peas	?
Mid-afternoon	?	?
Evening meal	?	?
During evening	Horlicks	?
Extras or during night	Tea with Maxijul Powder	50 ml

Figure 4.1 Poorly completed food chart

Day 2

Patient details: John Smith		Ward: B5
Time	Food/Drink	Quantity
Early morning	Cup of tea	180 ml
Breakfast	2 Weetabix with orange juice	Ate whole portion 100 ml
Mid-morning	Fortijuce	50 ml
Lunchtime	Cottage pie	Ate half a portion
	Peas	3 dessert spoons
	Glass of water	200 ml
	Cup of tea	180 ml
Mid-afternoon	Fortijuce	200 ml
Evening meal	Soup	Refused
	Cup of tea	180 ml
During evening	Horlicks	180 ml
Extras or during night	Water	100 ml

Figure 4.2 Accurately completed food chart showing measurable amounts of intake

Three to four days of measurable information recorded on a food chart will provide sufficient information to gain an indication of a patient's nutritional intake. Continuing to complete food charts over a longer period may result in poor completion and information being recorded inaccurately.

Use of specialised equipment

The use of appropriate specialised equipment to assist eating and drinking may prolong the patient's independence over their nutritional intake. Such equipment may include:

- non-slip mat: holds plates and glasses securely in place whilst eating and drinking
- plateguard: this may be useful for people who use one hand only when eating as it provides a wall at the edge of a plate against which the food can be pushed to manoeuvre it onto the spoon or fork
- adapted cutlery: cutlery can be adapted by using handgrips or holders designed to increase grip and function
- hands-free drinking equipment: this equipment is for users who are unable to lift and tilt a cup safely and/or cannot suck through a standard straw.

For more information, visit the Disabled Living Foundation's (2007) website at www.dlf.org.uk.

This type of equipment can be obtained following assessment from the occupational therapist. Although beneficial to some patients, adaptive cutlery is not always found on wards as it tends to either go missing or be left in meal trolleys making its use expensive.

Educating healthcare workers to assist patients with their meals

Educating healthcare staff to safely assist a patient to eat in a classroom environment can help them to gain an understanding of some of the difficulties that patients may experience in a hospital environment.

The following are examples of exercises that we have successfully used in teaching programmes. They can be a useful reminder of how it feels to be treated as a patient and not be in control of eating a meal or drinking independently and provide a base for further discussion.

These exercises tend to work better in smaller groups or pairs.

Prior to undertaking these exercises, check that none of the participants has an allergy to any of the ingredients used, for example Coeliac disease.

Exercise 1

For this exercise, get your participants to work in pairs. In turn, ask them to sit on their hands, close their eyes and try drinking water given in a plastic cup or glass by the second person. Get the second person to deliver the water slowly the first time whilst talking to the 'patient' and faster a second time without communicating.

Ask them to consider the following questions:

1. How does it feel?
2. Does the 'patient' feel safe/vulnerable?
3. How do they think patients on their ward may feel?
4. Highlight that for them this exercise is being carried out in a safe environment but the patient they will be caring for will be:
   ○ ill
   ○ apart from their family
   ○ in a strange environment
   ○ probably in their nightwear.

Get them to reflect upon how that may make their patients feel.

Exercise 2

Give each of your participants a small volume of a thickened drink.
Ask them to take note of how they feel when drinking it.
Discuss how it looks and tastes. Is it palatable?
Could you enhance the palatability of the drink?
How would you encourage your patient to drink it?

Remind them it is important to remember that the patient is likely to be influenced by the reaction of the nurse giving them their drink. Therefore it is important not to make negative responses regarding thickened drinks or supplements in front of the patient.

Exercise 3

Ask your students to try two nutrition supplement drinks, one that has been chilled in the fridge and a second at room temperature.
Get them to consider:

1. Which is more palatable and why?
2. Which drink would they normally offer to their patients?

Exercise 4

For this exercise, get your participants to work in pairs.
Ask the 'helper' to tell the 'patient' they will be receiving a particular food, e.g. strawberry-flavoured yoghurt, and then give them something different, e.g. a toffee-flavoured yoghurt or a biscuit, without communicating the change.
Ask the 'patient' how this feels.

References

Age Concern (2006) *Hungry to be Heard: The scandal of malnourished older people in hospital*, Age Concern, London.

Aronson, J.K. (2006) *Meyler's Side Effects of Drugs: The International Encyclopaedia of Adverse Drug Reactions & Interactions*, 15th edn, Elsevier, Oxford.

Association of Community Health Councils for England and Wales (1997) *Hungry in Hospital? Health News Briefing*, ACHCEW, London.

Bradley, L., Rees, C. (2003) Reducing nutritional risk in hospital: the red tray. *Nursing Standard* **17** (26), 33–7.

British Association for Parenteral and Enteral Nutrition (1999) *Hospital Food as Treatment: A report by a working party of the British Association for Parenteral and Enteral Nutrition*, BAPEN, Maidenhead.

Carr, E.K., Mitchell, J.R.A. (1991) A comparison of the mealtime care given to patients by nurses using two different meal delivery systems. *International Journal of Nursing Studies* **28** (1), 19–25.

Council of Europe (2002) *Food and nutritional care in hospitals: How to prevent under-nutrition: Report and recommendations of the Committee of Experts on Nutrition, Food Safety and Consumer Protection*, Council of Europe, Strasbourg.

Department of Health (1999) *Not Because They Are Old: An independent inquiry into the care of older people on acute wards in general hospitals*, Health Advisory Service 2000, DH, London.

Department of Health (2001a) *The Essence of Care: Patient-focused benchmarking for health care practitioners*, DH, London.

Department of Health (2001b) Health Circular HSC 20001/010 *Implementing the NHS Plan: Modern matrons*, DH, London.

Department of Health (2007) *Who Cares? Information and support for the carers of people with dementia*, DH, London.

Disabled Living Foundation (2007) http://www.dlf.org.uk, accessed 14 September 2007.

Hospital Caterers Association (2004) *Protected Mealtimes Policy*, HCA, London.

Hurley, A.C., Volicer, L. (2002) It's OK Mama if you want to go. It's OK. *Journal of the American Medical Association* **288**, 2324–31.

National Institute for Health and Clinical Excellence (2006) *Nutrition Support in Adults: Oral nutrition support, enteral tube feeding and parenteral nutrition, Clinical Guideline 32*, NICE, London.

NHS Estates (2001a) *Better Hospital Food Programme*, NHS Executive, London.

NHS Estates (2001b) Ward Housekeeping, http://patientexperience. nhsestates.gov.uk/ward_housekeeping/wh_content/home/home.asp, accessed 12 February 2008.

Royal College of Nursing (1993) *Nutritional Standards and the Older Adult: Dynamic Quality Improvement Programme*, RCN, London.

Royal College of Nursing (1996) *Statement on Feeding and Nutrition in Hospitals*, RCN, London.

Royal College of Nursing (2005) *Patients' Nutritional Care in Hospital: An ethnographic study of nurses' role and patients' experience*, RCN, London.

UK Central Council for Nursing, Midwifery and Health Visiting (1997) *Registrar's Letter: Responsibility for the feeding of patients*, UKCC, London.

Chapter 5

Enteral Nutrition

Carolyn Best, Helen Hitchings, Joanna Boult and Harriet Gordon

Introduction

Everyone needs food and water to stay alive and to keep their body functioning normally. A balanced diet is one that provides sufficient nutrients – energy, protein, vitamins and minerals – to keep an individual healthy.

Without an adequate balanced diet, an individual may not be receiving all the nutrients required for a healthy body. An inadequate diet can lead to malnutrition. Being malnourished can make you ill.

During illness, or following surgery, having an adequate and balanced diet is especially important. The body needs sufficient nutrients to aid recovery.

Undernourished individuals consume more healthcare resources (Martyn, 1998). It was estimated that in 2003 the annual cost of disease-related malnutrition in the United Kingdom was in excess of £7.3 billion (Elia *et al.*, 2005).

As previously seen in Chapter 1, there have been an array of documents and initiatives making recommendations to improve hospital food – from improving access to food and food provision to identifying those needing help with food and food presentation, including *Hospital Food as Treatment* (Allison, 1999), *Better Hospital Food: The NHS Plan* (Department of Health, 2000), *Essence of Care: Patient-focused benchmarking* (Department of Health, 2001) and *Improving Nutritional Care* (Department of Health, 2007).

Following screening and assessment, if the need for nutritional support is identified, the next step in the process is to decide which form of nutrition support would be the most appropriate.

If an individual is capable of eating, yet is unable to consume sufficient nutrition, there is a stepwise fashion for escalating nutrition support:

1. Snacks
2. Fortified foods
3. Sip feeds
4. Short-term enteral feeding
5. Long-term enteral feeding

So, the first line in nutritional support would be to provide additional drinks and snacks between meals. If, once established, this form of support is insufficient, the next step would be to offer fortified foods and drinks. If this still provides insufficient nutrients, sip feeds may be commenced. If, even with the introduction of sip feeds, the patient's oral intake remains suboptimal, or the individual is unable to swallow safely, short-term enteral feeding would be the next step. If this is in addition to oral intake, this may be given overnight, or in bolus feeds during the day. If an individual is unable to consume any oral intake, this may be given in a continual manner throughout the day.

The next sections will elaborate on this incremental approach to increasing nutrition.

Oral nutrition support

As already discussed, the oral route is the route of choice when aiming to increase nutritional intake: if the gut works, use it!

Appropriate diet

In practice, initially, something as basic as ensuring that people have something to eat at least three times a day can be beneficial. Then look at what is being eaten. Is sufficient protein being consumed? Is the person on an appropriate diet – or are they on a 'low calorie', 'weight reducing'-type diet, with low-sugar/low-fat food and drinks? Ensuring people are having enough of the right food to eat should be the first step. If they are able to manage a higher oral intake between meals, snacks (such as cheese and biscuits, a yoghurt or a sandwich) can be introduced to significantly add to a day's total calorie intake. It is essential that these snacks are in addition to, and not in place of, meals; so they need to be presented well before the next meal is due. If the patient is able to manage more food at meal-times, increasing the size of their portions may help to increase their overall intake. Often, it is easier to eat more if foods are not too high in fibre – as fibre can make people feel full. Ensuring that individuals are not constipated may help too: there is nothing like constipation for dulling an appetite. For people with wounds or pressure ulcers, protein intake is important, but it is also essential that the individual has sufficient energy to enable the body to utilise the protein efficiently. Otherwise, the dietary protein is just used as an energy source for the body.

So our suggested action plan would be:

- **Normal diet:** increase portions where appropriate/possible.
- **High-energy/high-protein diet:** with appropriately coded menus and advice from qualified professionals.
- **Between-meals snacks:** in addition to meals, a little and often approach – not always easy with in-patients.
- **Between-meals nutritious drinks:** for individuals with poor appetites, it is often easier to drink a nutritious drink than it is to be faced with another meal or snack. Drinks can be anything from milky coffee or hot chocolate to milk or milkshake, or a soup. Generally, drinks based on milk are more nutritious than those based on water. Aim to maximise an individual's intake by not allowing them to fill themselves by drinking vast quantities of plain water before or during a meal.

In healthy adults, the World Health Organization (WHO; 2002) recommends 1 g/kg/day protein. In illness, protein intake often falls just when protein requirements often increase to 1.2–2.5 g/kg/day (Elia, 1996; Soulsby & Weekes, 2004). This can result in a protein gap of 40 g/day.

Additional food, snacks and drinks may not be to everyone's taste, and so the next step is to fortify foods.

Fortifying foods

Quite simply, this is preferable because it is often more acceptable for the patient to receive fortified food, which may still appear normal and be more palatable, than needing to rely on supplements. It may also be of benefit psychologically to be able to consume normal food, rather than needing to rely on oral nutritional supplements or tube feeding (Mahan & Arlin, 1992).

Most catering departments are capable of providing fortified foods – for example mashed potato with added skimmed-milk powder, milk with additional milk powder – to supply additional protein and calories (energy).

The liberal addition of cream, butter, full-cream milk, dried-milk powder and grated cheese can add significantly to the overall daily energy and protein intake.

It is easy to fortify many soft/moist foods with either additional protein or energy, or both, for example grated cheese in mashed potato.

Oral nutritional supplements

If the provision of additional food, snacks or fortified food proves to be insufficient, or not well tolerated, the next step would be to try to introduce nutritional supplements – either food or drinks that have been artificially created to be as nutrient-dense as possible in order to maximise an individual's intake. These supplements come in several forms, although the most common tend to be the nutritionally complete liquids provided in cartons or bottles, for example Fortisip, Ensure, Clinutren and Resource. The use of nutritionally complete supplements can be used to improve an individual's nutritional intake and consequently nutritional status. 'Nutritionally complete' means that if sufficient quantities of the supplement are consumed an individual's theoretical nutritional requirements for all vitamins and minerals, energy and protein can be met. They are not, however, nutritionally complete in one bottle or carton. A dietitian should advise how many supplements are required in order to meet a patient's nutritional requirements.

There tend to be three main options for these drinks:

- milkshake style 1 kcal/ml or high-energy 1.5 kcal/ml with or without fibre
- fruit juice style 1.5 kcal/ml
- yogurt style 1.5 kcal/ml.

The milkshake and fruit juice style supplements tend to be fairly sweet (there are a few savoury flavours available), whilst the yoghurt style drinks are less so. Also, providing a combination of the different types of supplements works well, because combinations prevent taste fatigue. Often, individuals who are malnourished or unwell do have taste changes; so it is as well to offer a range of different flavours when establishing which drinks will be tolerated.

Other powdered supplements that can be made into milkshake style drinks with fresh milk include Build-up, Complan, Calshake, Enshake, Foodlink Complete and Scandishake Mix. These may be more palatable for some as they are made with fresh milk, and consequently taste fresher and more like a milkshake.

There are also savoury soup type supplements that are presented in powdered form, for example Vegenat Med and Vitasavoury.

There are semisolid type 'puddings', such as Forticreme Complete, Clinutren Dessert, Formance, Resource Energy Dessert and Fortipudding.

Other supplements available include:

- **completely fat-based liquid:** either flavoured to drink on its own or unflavoured to be used in cooking (Calogen), e.g. in porridge
- **carbohydrate and fat:** Duocal, as liquid emulsion, or Super Soluble Powder
- **pure carbohydrate powder:** Maxijul Super Soluble, Vitajoule, Caloreen and Polycose (this is unflavoured and easily dissolvable and so can be added to drinks and moist foods to provide additional energy)
- **pure carbohydrate liquid:** Polycal, Maxijul (flavoured or unflavoured); this supplement can be drunk although is sometimes better diluted with something like lemonade, otherwise it's rather like drinking syrup
- **protein powder:** Maxipro, Vitapro, Protifar, dried milk powder
- **protein and energy powder:** Procal or QuickCal can be added to a range of sweet and savoury dishes to provide additional nutrients. It contains protein, fat and carbohydrate
- **MCT (medium-chain triglycerides) fat supplementation:** Liquigen, useful in patients with steatorrhoea, in chronic liver disease/cirrhosis, proven malabsorption.

These supplements tend not to be nutritionally complete; so they are beneficial in providing additional energy or protein, but they may not provide all vitamins and minerals, unlike the nutritionally complete drinks.

With all types of oral nutrition support, monitoring is essential. Intake charts accurately completed, by the patient concerned where possible, or care staff, are invaluable in assessing the nutritional value of oral intake. Together with daily oral intake charts, the patient requiring a supplemented diet should be weighed initially as a baseline, and then weekly to monitor progress.

Box 5.1   Potential complications which may arise during the intubation procedure

---

- Damage to the nasal mucosa
- Intracranial intubation
- Curling of the tube in the patient's mouth
- Pharyngeal or oesophageal pouch perforation
- Bronchial placement

Options for enteral tube feeding: short-term feeding

Nasogastric feeding

A nasogastric tube is the most common method of providing access for short-term enteral feeding. It provides the means by which a nutritionally adequate diet can be provided directly into the stomach, bypassing the oral route.

Patient assessment

Before intubation of a nasogastric tube is attempted, the nurse must be aware of possible complications associated with the procedure (Box 5.1). A detailed patient history should be obtained to identify any problems that would make intubation technically difficult or even impossible, such as previous nasal fractures or surgery, nasal polyps or other blockages. The nurse should be aware of the rationale for nasogastric feeding and of the projected period for which this feeding will be required. This may affect the type and size of the nasogastric feeding tube selected. Nasogastric feeding is usually used in patients who require short-term enteral feeding, i.e. four to six weeks, and have a functioning gastrointestinal tract. There are cases where nasogastric feeding is continued for longer than the four to six weeks recommended, for example patient preference or where alternative methods of providing enteral feeding are difficult or unsafe. Obviously, where a nasogastric tube is used for longer periods, there is an increased risk of the patient developing ulceration along the nasal passages and oesophagus.

Although the most common method of providing short-term enteral nutrition, nasogastric feeding is not a suitable option for all patients. Care should be taken when considering this method of feeding with patients who have:

- a high risk of aspiration
- gastro-oesophageal reflux

- upper-gastrointestinal-tract disease
- base of skull fractures
- poor gastric emptying, a suspected ileus or intestinal obstruction.

Where these complications exist or if a long-term feeding option is required, other routes of enteral feeding should be considered.

Choosing a tube

A fine-bore nasogastric tube should be used in preference to a wide-bore or Ryle's tube for enteral feeding. The fine-bore is a more comfortable option for the patient and minimises the risk of developing rhinitis, pharyngitis or oesophageal erosion. Dewar (1997) recommends the use of a 6 fr (ch) tube with a minimum length of 90 cm, whilst Rollins (1997) suggests that standard feeds can be administered through a 6 fr (ch) tube with ease but an 8 fr (ch) may be required for patients receiving a fibre feed. NICE (2006) recommends 5–8 fr (ch).

Fine-bore nasogastric tubes are made from either polyvinylchloride (PVC) or polyurethane. The former is used for enteral feeding required for only seven to 10 days. Beyond this period, the PVC tube begins to break down as the chemical plasticisers designed to keep the tube flexible gradually leach out, leaving the tube brittle and at risk of cracking. This rigidity increases the risk of the patient developing nasal or oesophageal erosion. A polyurethane tube is not affected in the same way and remains soft and flexible throughout use. It is therefore not surprisingly the tube of choice for most patients.

When making the decision of what type of nasogastric tube to use, a number of issues need to be considered. The nasogastric tube should be radio-opaque and have clear centimetre or line markers to aid measurement during the intubation procedure and bedside checks.

Additional factors to consider include:

- size fr (ch) and internal lumen of the tube
- length
- ease of intubation
- number of ports and exit points
- ease of aspiration/flushing
- type of feed to be administered
- patient comfort/preference
- cost.

Preparation of the patient

The patient should be in a semi-upright position in a bed or chair. The head should be supported with pillows (Dougherty & Lister, 2008) and not tilted forwards or backwards (Rollins, 1997). If the patient cannot sit upright, the procedure can be carried out by laying the patient on their side (Bowling, 2004).

The proposed procedure should be clearly explained to the patient, avoiding the use of jargon, and their role within it clarified. Agree a signal, such as the raising of a hand so that the patient retains some control over the situation and may stop the procedure at any time if they feel uncomfortable or unsafe. The patient's verbal consent must be obtained before the procedure is attempted. Where this is not possible, for example in a patient who is unconscious or unable to make an informed decision, discussions should be held with all relevant healthcare professionals involved in the patient's care to ensure that a nasogastric tube intubation is in the best interests of the patient.

Agree with the patient into which nostril the nasogastric tube is to be inserted. Where possible, each nostril should be used alternately if repeated nasogastric tube intubations are necessary. Ask the patient to blow their nose to clear their nasal passages and check the oral cavity is clear. Finally, where appropriate, provide the patient with a glass of water.

Box 5.2 lists the equipment necessary to undertake nasogastric tube intubation.

Procedure

The intubation of a nasogastric tube should only be attempted a maximum of three times by one individual. If intubation is still

Box 5.2   Equipment required for nasogastric tube intubation

Fine-bore nasogastric tube
50 ml syringe
pH indicator strips
Receiver
Lubricating jelly (if required)
Glass of water with drinking straw (if patient not nil by mouth)
Tissues
Hypoallergenic tape and scissors
Freshly run tap water from a drinking source, for flushing
Non-sterile gloves and apron

unsuccessful after the third attempt, seek assistance (Cannaby *et al.*, 2002).

The following provides a step-by-step guide to nasogastric tube intubation:

1. This is a clean procedure; so gloves and apron should be worn.
2. Remove nasogastric tube from packaging, stretching gently to remove any kinks or bends.
3. Ensure guide wire is firmly secured at the tip of the tube.
4. Check that all access ports are closed.
5. Estimate the length of nasogastric tube to be advanced into the patient. This measurement is used to provide an indication of when the tube reaches the stomach. To estimate the length of tube required, hold the proximal (stomach) end of the nasogastric tube loosely at the tip of the patient's nose. Extend the tube to the earlobe and down to the xiphoid process. At this point, the closest depth mark on the tube should be noted or the tube marked directly with a pen (Burnham, 2000).
6. Activate the lubricant at the tip of the tube by dipping the end in freshly run tap water. Although not always necessary, additional lubricating jelly can be used, if required.
7. Gently insert the tip of the nasogastric tube into the agreed nostril, sliding it slowly backwards, not upwards, along the floor of the nasopharynx and into the back of the mouth.
8. Never advance the tube against any resistance.
9. Stop immediately if the patient begins to cough, has difficulty breathing or becomes cyanosed.
10. If there are no signs of distress, ask the patient to breathe through their mouth and swallow when they feel the tube at the back of their throat. As the patient swallows gently advance the tube through the oesophagus and into the stomach. If the patient can drink a sip of water, encourage them to do so as it may help them swallow the tube at this point.
11. Continue passing the tube until the measured depth mark is reached. Do not push the nasogastric tube beyond the agreed depth mark.
12. Secure tube loosely to nose or cheek.
13. Confirm the position of the tube. Do not remove the guide wire before the final position of the tip of the tube is confirmed. Repositioning a nasogastric tube without a guide wire can be quite difficult and attempts to reinsert the guide wire whilst the nasogastric tube is in the patient exposes the patient to potential harm.

Confirming position

The nurse inserting the nasogastric tube is responsible for confirming that the tip is situated in the stomach before commencing a feed regimen or administering medications. Incorrect positioning in the bronchial tract or oesophagus could result in aspiration of feed or fluid. In the *Patient Safety Alert* published in February 2005, the National Patient Safety Agency (NPSA) cited 11 deaths and one case of serious harm, over a two-year period, due to misplaced nasogastric tubes.

Historically, nurses have used a number of different methods to confirm nasogastric tube position, some of which in recent years have been shown to be unsafe (Box 5.3). In an attempt to minimise the risk of injury caused by misplaced tubes, the NPSA (2005) has produced guidelines indicating which methods for checking tube position should be used: gastric aspirate and abdominal X-ray.

Any incident involving the feeding of a patient via an incorrectly positioned nasogastric tube should be reported to clinical governance as a clinical incident.

Methods of confirming tube position

The initial tube position must be confirmed using one of the following methods:

- aspiration of gastric contents
- X-ray.

Aspiration of gastric contents   Testing gastric aspirate with pH indicator strips should be the first method used to confirm tube position on initial placement. Although many tales abound to the contrary, it is possible to aspirate gastric contents through a fine-bore nasogastric tube with the guide wire still in situ.

To reduce any potential problems during the checking procedure:

- ensure all access ports are closed before attaching a 50 ml syringe to the main feeding port
- inject a small amount of air into the tube to clear the exit points of debris and move the tip of the tube away from the gastric mucosa.

Using the same 50 ml syringe, aspirate a specimen of stomach contents back through the tube gently. Less than 1 ml of aspirate is sufficient to check tube position (National Patient Safety Agency, 2005). It

Box 5.3 Unsafe methods of confirming tube position

The 'whoosh' test

This involves the insufflation of air into the nasogastric tube while a second person listens with a stethoscope over the abdomen for a distinctive 'whooshing' sound. Metheny *et al.* (1990) clearly highlight the difficulty in differentiating between lung, oesophageal or gastric placement, as the sound emitted is generalised over the abdomen.

Observing for air bubbles

The proximal end of the tube is placed under water and observed for air bubbles. The assumption is that if the tube has been placed in the lungs the bubbles will be seen on expiration (Colagiovanni, 1999). However, gas bubbles may be produced in the stomach. Reliance on this method could falsely indicate respiratory placement (Metheny & Meert, 2004) and may result in a correctly positioned tube being needlessly removed.

Absence of respiratory distress

Respiratory symptoms are less likely to occur with the use of small-bore polyurethane tubes. However, the absence of respiratory distress should not be interpreted as an indicator of correct positioning. Patients who are unconscious or do not have an effective gag reflex will not necessarily exhibit the signs of coughing or cyanosis expected with intubation into the bronchial tract even if, in some cases, a large-bore tube is used.

Blue litmus paper

The use of blue litmus paper to check the acidity of aspirate is now recognised as being insufficiently sensitive to distinguish between the required level of acidity. This is because it changes colour in the presence of acid rather than defining the exact pH value (Khair, 2005). Therefore, a bronchial placement with a pH of 6 will still indicate acidity on litmus paper, leading to the possible use of an incorrectly placed nasogastric tube, with disastrous consequences. The Medicines and Healthcare products Regulatory Agency (MHRA; 2004) issued an alert in June 2004 advising all staff to stop using blue litmus paper to test the acidity/alkalinity of aspirate.

Observing the colour of feeding tube aspirate without checking its pH

Metheny *et al.* (1994) examined the gastric aspirate of 880 patients. They established that gastric aspirates ranged in colour from green, yellow, tan, brown to bloody, while respiratory aspirate was similarly described as tan or yellow/green. With such variable results, this measure cannot reliably be used to determine tube placement.

is important to note that it may take more than one attempt to aspirate gastric fluid, particularly if the patient has not received nutrition for over a week, but be prepared to persevere if unsuccessful first time round.

The size and length of the nasogastric tube used may influence the ability of the nurse to aspirate gastric contents. Aspiration is easier with an 8 fr (ch) tube than with a 6 fr (ch) and with the shorter 90–95 cm tubes rather than the longer 110 cm tubes.

Once aspirate is obtained, test its acidity with pH-specific indicator strips. A pH of 0–5.5 indicates gastric placement. For patients receiving acid-inhibiting drugs, Metheny *et al.* (1993, 1994) recorded pH readings of between 4 to 6, but in practice most patients still have a pH of less than 5.5.

Bronchial placement should be suspected if the aspirate has a pH of 6–8 (Metheny *et al.*, 1993, 1994; Colagiovanni, 1999), even if the signs of respiratory distress are not always present. Intestinal placement is indicated with a pH of 5–6. It is worth noting that the feed itself can increase the pH in the stomach; so, if there is a need to check tube position once a feed has been commenced, stop the feed and aspirate at least one hour after the feed has been stopped (National Institute for Health and Clinical Excellence, 2006).

TROUBLESHOOTING TIPS
The most common problems associated with not being able to obtain aspirate include:

- one of the tube's ports remains open
- the tube is not situated in a pocket of fluid.

If problems are experienced, have patience and try working through the following measures:

(NB: The administration of air into a nasogastric tube suggested in these tips is not intended to confirm position by listening to bubbles over the abdomen, i.e. the 'whoosh' test.)

- Inject 10 ml of air into the tube. If the patient belches, the tip of the nasogastric tube is probably sitting in the oesophagus (Metheny *et al.*, 1993, 1994). Advance the tube and repeat the aspirate test.

- The nasogastric tube may be situated in the air space above the aspirate level in the stomach. Advance the tube 5–10 cm and repeat the aspirate test.
- The tip of the tube may be sitting against the gastric mucosa. Inject 10 ml of air into the stomach to push the port away from the gastric mucosa and clear any debris. Repeat the aspirate test.
- If intestinal placement is suspected, withdraw the tube 5–10 cm and repeat the aspirate test.
- If the patient shows signs of respiratory distress or the aspirate is pH 6–8, remove the tube and re-pass.
  (NB: Not all patients will show signs of respiratory distress even when the tube is in the bronchial tract.)
- If aspirate is still not obtained, lay the patient on his or her left side, wait one hour (National Institute for Health and Clinical Excellence, 2006) and attempt aspiration again. The change in position will allow the fluid level in the stomach to move, making aspiration easier.

Aspiration of visually recognisable gastric contents This method of confirmation can only be used in patients who have an intact swallow and are able to take a drink orally. The patient is asked to drink a visually identifiable liquid, such as milk or blackcurrant juice. If the fluid can then be aspirated back up through the nasogastric tube, gastric placement is indicated.

X-ray Radiography is not recommended as a routine method for checking nasogastric tube position (National Institute for Health and Clinical Excellence, 2006). Therefore, this method should only be used to confirm the positioning of the tip of the tube on initial placement. It is important to remember that an X-ray will only confirm the position of the tip of the nasogastric tube at the time the X-ray is carried out. By the time the patient has left the medical imaging department and returned to the ward, the nasogastric tube may have become displaced. For this reason, other methods for checking tube position must be used at the bedside, i.e. aspirate checks.

Your local policy will indicate precisely when an X-ray should be used, but guidance may indicate its use for patients who are:

- unconscious
- on a ventilator

or when

- after repeated attempts, no aspirate has been obtained
- the pH of aspirate obtained is >5.5.

Capnography   Capnography is a method of detecting carbon dioxide (CO_2) levels and is used to highlight possible inadvertent bronchial placement. The nasogastric tube is inserted to approximately 30–35 cm and a detector secured onto the end of the nasogastric tube. A small bellows is attached to the detector and air is sucked through the system. If the detector changes colour, the presence of CO_2 is indicated, suggesting that the nasogastric tube is sitting in the bronchial tract. This system provides a clear visual indication of tube position and acts to minimise patient trauma by blind advancement of a tube into the bronchial tract. This method of monitoring is currently in its infancy but may have a bigger part to play in the future.

Following confirmation of tube position

Once tube placement is confirmed, the guide wire can be removed and the tube flushed with 20–30 ml of water to clear it of debris built up during the intubation procedure. The guide wire must not be reinserted into the nasogastric tube whilst the tube remains in the patient.

Some hospitals may recommend keeping the guide wire at the bedside for 24 hours in a plastic bag labelled with the patient's name, hospital number and date of intubation in case repositioning is necessary. In reality, this could be considered an infection risk. It is probably just as easy to intubate the patient with a new tube.

Securing the tube

The risk of displacement of a nasogastric tube is relatively high. Patients may inadvertently knock the tube or attempt to pull it, resulting in the dislodgement into the oesophagus, increasing the risk of aspiration or regurgitation. Tube position may also change following episodes of coughing, retching or vomiting. Metheny *et al.* (1986) report that 15% of nasogastric tubes became displaced following confirmation of initial placement without the nursing staff being aware of this happening. This highlights the need for continued routine bedside monitoring of tube position (Box 5.4).

Nasogastric tubes should be taped securely at the nose to avoid inadvertent displacement and in a manner that is acceptable to the

Box 5.4 When to check nasogastric tube placement

Tube position must be checked:

- on initial placement
- before the administration of feed following a break or when bolus feeding
- before the administration of drugs if the tube is not used for any other purpose
- after episodes of coughing, retching or vomiting
- after the use of oropharyngeal suction
- if the tube appears to have changed in length
- at least once daily during continuous feeds
- if the patient complains of discomfort or feed reflux into the throat or mouth
- if the patient suddenly has signs of respiratory difficulties, including breathlessness, stridor, cyanosis or wheezing
- if the patient is transferred from one clinical area to another, the receiving clinical area must verify tube position before commencing a feed.

Additional monitoring techniques

- Mark the tube with an indelible pen at the nostril.
- Record the length of the tube at the point of exit from the nostril.
- Perform daily checks of nasal-fixation tapes.
- Check for signs of respiratory discomfort or regurgitation (not always present).

(NB: All actions to monitor tube position should be documented in the patient's notes.)

patient. Some companies supply a plaster with the tube, but for those that do not the use of a soft pliable tape is recommended.

If the patient has oily skin or perspires readily, the adhesive tapes may need regular replacement. In such cases, the use of an alcohol wipe to clean the skin and an adhesive dressing may be of use. Once secure at the nose, the remaining length of tube should be loosely taped to the cheek, out of the patient's vision and tucked behind their ear when not in use.

Where there is a risk of tube displacement, the use of a nasal bridle or loop may be appropriate. It may also prove useful where there are technical difficulties in placement and the tube has to be retained for as long as possible or where there is a need to maintain access whilst decisions are made regarding longer-term feeding options. This method has been used with positive results in both dysphasic and critically ill patients with minimal rates of complication (Popovich *et al.*, 1996; Anderson *et al.*, 2004).

This device secures the nasogastric tube at the nose using a length of umbilical tape. Using magnets placed at the end of two probes, a length of umbilical tape is passed through the patient's nostrils and behind the nasal septum and is then drawn through so that one end of the tape sits in both nostrils. The tape is tied and, along with the nasogastric tube, secured in a plastic clip directly below one nostril.

Nasojejunal feeding

Nasojejunal feeding is a short-term option for providing enteral nutrition into the gastrointestinal tract, bypassing the stomach and feeding directly into the small intestine (post-pyloric feeding).

It is suitable for patients with:

- gastroparesis
- pancreatitis
- an increased risk of aspiration associated with gastric feeding.

Nasojejunal tubes

Nasojejunal (NJ) tubes come with a number of different features, including:

- weighted and non-weighted tips
- pigtails
- single- or double-lumen.

Unweighted vs weighted tips

Weighted tubes were introduced with the aim that the extra weight in the tip of the tube would help to retain the position of the tube in the small intestine. In our experience, they are often no more effective than non-weighted tubes.

Single- and double-lumen tubes

A single-lumen tube placed in the jejunum can be successful in providing enteral nutrition, but where there is an ongoing problem with gastric emptying, for example in the critically ill patient, the use of a double-lumen NJ tube may be appropriate. This will provide a gastric port for the aspiration of gastric contents and a jejunal port for feeding. A double-lumen tube is slightly larger in diameter than the single-lumen tube and may therefore be more uncomfortable for the patient. However, it is worth bearing in mind that it is still a better option than two single-lumen tubes – one for aspiration and one for feeding, in either nostril.

Patient assessment

This is as per nasogastric tubes.

Potential complications

- as per nasogastric tubes
- difficult placement
- migration of the tip of the tube back into the stomach; as there is no means of securing the NJ tube internally, this can be a fairly common problem

Passing a nasojejunal tube

These tubes can be placed either endoscopically, radiologically or at the bedside using prokinetic drugs to stimulate gastric emptying.

Bedside placement

The Bengmark (Nutricia) or Corpak (Merck) tubes are designed to be passed at the bedside. These tubes are inserted into the stomach as per the nasogastric tube. Once gastric positioning is confirmed using gastric aspirate or X-ray, further passage of the tube through the pylorus is encouraged by utilising normal gastric motility or, where this is insufficient, via the addition of a prokinetic agent such as metoclopramide. The Bengmark tube has a 'pigtail' or 'spiral' to assist gastroduodenal motility (see below).

To ensure a continued gradual movement of the tube through the pylorus during the intubation procedure, the NJ tube should only be loosely secured at the cheek or tucked behind the ear. It must not be firmly attached to the nose at this stage as this will inhibit tube migration into the small intestine. This final stage of tube positioning may take between anything from six to 24 hours to achieve.

Final placement of an NJ tube placed at the bedside must be verified by abdominal X-ray before feeding can commence.

This method may not be effective in some critically ill patients where gastric motility is impaired or for those taking prescribed sedative agents, such as morphine (Davies *et al.*, 2002). Using endoscopic or radiological placement may be a better option for these patients.

Endoscopic placement of a nasojejunal tube

As with any endoscopic procedure, the patient should be counselled and consented prior to the endoscopic placement of an NJ tube. The patient is admitted to endoscopy and sedated appropriately. The endoscope is placed through the oral cavity into the stomach and through into the duodenum, and then advanced as far as possible distally. The NJ tube is then advanced through the biopsy channel of the endoscope into the duodenum under direct observation. Once the NJ tube reaches the duodenum, the endoscope is carefully removed leaving the NJ tube in situ. The NJ tube is now jejunum to mouth so needs re-routing to the nose. To do this, a re-routing catheter is used. The re-routing catheter is advanced through the nasal passages into the pharynx, and then brought out through the mouth using Magill forceps and a laryngoscope. It is then lubricated and the end of the NJ tube attached to it. Finally, the re-routing catheter and tip of the NJ tube is pulled out through the nose. The tube is now nasojejunal. The final placement of the NJ tube must be confirmed by X-ray.

Radiological placement of a nasojejunal tube

The radiological placement of an NJ tube is not dissimilar to an endoscopic placement. Insertion of the tube is initially via the nose. Screening is used to check the correct passage as the tube is passed down the oesophagus, through the stomach and duodenum and into the proximal jejunum. Manual dexterity is required to manoeuvre the tube through the pylorus and beyond. Once in place, the guide wire is removed.

Securing the tube

Once tube position has been confirmed, secure as per nasogastric tube.

Options for enteral tube feeding: long-term feeding

Patients who require enteral feeding extending beyond six weeks require a more permanent means of access than either a nasogastric or NJ tube can offer. A gastrostomy tube is the most common means of providing this. A gastrostomy tube provides access directly into the stomach through the development of a fistula through the abdomen.

Gastric feeding

There are a number of different intubation techniques and gastrostomy tubes available. These include:

- the percutaneous endoscopic gastrostomy (PEG)
- a radiologically inserted gastrostomy (RIG) or fluoroscopically guided percutaneous gastrostomy (FPG)
- the balloon gastrostomy (also called a 'replacement gastrostomy' or 'G tube')
- the button or low-profile device
- surgical intubation: may involve insertion of any of the above tubes.

Percutaneous endoscopic gastrostomy

A percutaneous endoscopic gastrostomy (PEG) tube is the most frequently used method of gastrostomy insertion. The tubes are usually made from polyurethane and are therefore fairly resilient, lasting for up to a couple of years. They are retained in the stomach by a small disc, flange or cone-shaped device and held externally by a movable fixation device or bolster. There are a number of contraindications and complications associated with a PEG insertion procedure (Table 5.1)

Table 5.1 Complications and contraindications to PEG insertion

Complications	Contraindications
Early (<30 days):	A PEG is not appropriate for patients who:
• bowel perforation • haemorrhage • peritonitis • aspiration	• are obese (as transillumination and accessing the stomach safely will be difficult) • have breathing difficulties (if the patient cannot lie relatively flat for 20–30 minutes for the procedure to take place) • have an uncorrected coagulopathy (patient should have a normal INR) • have gastric ulcers • have a gastric malignancy • have had a gastrectomy.

that may necessitate the need to seek an alternative means of providing access.

Radiologically inserted gastrostomy

Where endoscopic placement is difficult or contraindicated, a gastrostomy may be placed under radiological guidance. This technique requires insufflation of the stomach through a nasogastric tube and external puncture of the abdomen. These tubes usually have a shorter lifespan than a PEG and may be removed once the stoma tract has matured to be replaced with a button or balloon gastrostomy.

They are held in the abdomen by a flexible loop, or pigtail, formed by pulling of a length of cotton string that travels along the inner length of the tube to be wound around and secured at the distal end of the tube. This forms the internal retention device. Should the cotton string break or be dislodged, the pigtail is released and there is nothing holding the tube in place internally, and it is therefore at a greater risk of falling out.

Surgical insertion of a gastrostomy

Since the introduction of endoscopic placement of gastrostomies, this technique is used less frequently in adults. It tends to be used where other techniques have proved unsuccessful or where the patient has anatomical abnormalities, for example a patient with a hiatus hernia. Here, using a laparoscopic approach, the stomach is pulled down using atraumatic forceps and stitched to the anterior abdominal wall. Once secure, a PEG can be placed using an endoscope in the usual manner.

Balloon

A balloon gastrostomy, or G tube, is used as a replacement gastrostomy into a mature tract following the primary insertion of a PEG or RIG. It may also be used for a primary placement using surgical insertion. It is held in place in the stomach via a balloon inflated with water and usually has a lifespan of approximately three to six months. One advantage of using this type of gastrostomy in a mature tract is that tube changes are percutaneous and therefore less invasive than endoscopic replacement and can be carried out at the patient's bedside in a hospital or within their own home.

Button

A button gastrostomy, or low-profile/skin-level device, is usually placed percutaneously in a mature stoma tract. It is held in place by a water balloon or traction removal device. It has an anti-reflux valve designed to prevent the backflow of stomach contents through the top of the tube. An extension set is attached to the 'button' during feeding, which can be easily removed.

To ensure the correct fitting of a button gastrostomy, it is essential that the stoma tract is measured in both diameter and length before a tube is placed to minimise the development of potential complications.

These tubes are useful in patients:

- who require a more discreet and less obtrusive device, for cosmetic reasons. It can be worn under tighter clothing or sportswear and is therefore more compatible for younger, more ambulant patients
- for whom frequent gastrostomy tube changes are to be avoided. It is durable and tends to last longer than balloon gastrostomy tubes
- who have a tendency to pull at their gastrostomy tube. Self-extubation is more difficult than with standard gastrostomy tubes.

Insertion of both the balloon and button gastrostomies can be done at the bedside or in the patient's own home.

Jejunal feeding

Percutaneous endoscopic gastrojejunostomy

A percutaneous endoscopic gastrojejunostomy (PEGJ) is used for long-term post-pyloric enteral feeding. Indications for the use of this type of feeding tube are as for an NJ tube. A PEGJ is created with the primary placement of a PEG. Once in place, a long, small-gauge tube is passed through the lumen of the PEG and is pulled down into the small intestine with the assistance of endoscopic forceps.

Unfortunately, there is a risk of the jejunal tube being dislodged as the endoscope is withdrawn from the small intestine. It is essential to monitor the length of the tubing advanced into the small intestine during the insertion procedure as the introduction of excess tubing is likely to do more harm than good. It may result in the extension tubing curling up in the stomach causing knotting or retrograde movement of the tip into the stomach.

As with a nasogastric tube, the jejunal extension is not secured internally. It is only attached to the PEG at the external tip of the tube. It is important to note that, although it may appear bulky, all the attachments at the distal end of the tubing are required. They are integral to ensuring the jejunal tube is safely secured. Unscrewing or trying to remove any part of these attachments may lead to misplacement of the jejunal tube either by accidentally pulling the jejunal extension out of the PEG or by dislodging it from its means of attachment, allowing it to loosen and travel down the internal lumen of the PEG as water or feed is administered through the end of the tube. Although rare, if not detected, the jejunal extension may partially or completely advance into the stomach where it will curl up completely or if the tip remains in the jejunum, with the assistance of peristalsis, result in spontaneous rectal expulsion. Often, misplacement is only identified when the patient complains of symptoms such as nausea or starts vomiting.

Radiologically inserted gastrojejunostomy

Inserted as per an RIG.

Surgically placed needle catheter jejunostomy

This is placed directly into the jejunum at laparotomy. The method of securement is dependent upon the manufacturer. Some surgical jejunostomies are tunnelled and are secured using a Dacron cuff, whilst others are only held in place by sutures at the abdomen.

Patient assessment and preparation

Endoscopic, radiological or surgical intubation techniques

A detailed patient history should be obtained before the patient is sent for primary placement of a gastrostomy tube, to ensure that they are medically stable to undergo the procedure and that the insertion of a gastrostomy is appropriate for their needs. The proposed procedure and aftercare required should be discussed with the patient and their relatives and carers.

The type of tube to be used will be decided upon following discussion with the patient and others involved in their care, and a written information sheet should be provided to back up discussions. Written informed consent must be obtained from the patient. If the patient is unable to sign their own consent form, this must be documented and consent obtained from the patient's medical lead in their best interest.

The patient should be fasted for six hours prior to a PEG or RIG insertion, but clear fluids may usually be given up to two hours before the procedure. If the patient is receiving anticoagulation therapy, it may need to be stopped approximately four to five days before the procedure and the patient's INR checked.

Percutaneous balloon/button gastrostomy changes

The decision to change to a balloon or button gastrostomy will usually be made by the patient's gastroenterologist, nutrition nurse specialist or Nutrition Team in conjunction with the patient. They will only be placed into a mature tract. Feeding via the gastrostomy should be stopped a couple of hours prior to the tube change.

Aftercare of gastrostomy tubes

The percutaneous endoscopic gastrostomy tube

1. The patient should remain nil by mouth (NBM) and nil by tube for four hours (National Institute for Health and Clinical Excellence, 2006).
2. Baseline observations should be checked as the patient has undergone an invasive procedure requiring sedation. Temperature, pulse, respiration and blood pressure should be monitored regularly during the first 24 hours to monitor for signs of possible complications (Table 5.2).
3. After four hours, the tube should be flushed with 30–50 ml of water (freshly run tap, cooled boiled or sterile – according to local guidelines) to assess patient comfort. If the patient feels no discomfort and there is no resistance to the flush, the feeding regimen can commence as per dietetic guidelines.

Table 5.2 Post PEG insertion observations

Observations	Timings
Temperature, pulse and respiration (TPR) and blood pressure	Every 30 minutes for the first four hours
	Hourly for two hours
	Six-hourly (QDS) for at least the next 24 hours

4. For the first week to 10 days, the PEG site should be cleaned with normal saline and sterile gauze at least once a day using an aseptic technique. The sides of the external fixation device should be lifted to check the skin around the stoma site for erythema, tenderness, irritation and discharge. Refer to local guidelines for type of dressing used.
5. Do not tape the PEG tube to the abdomen for the first two weeks, to encourage straight stoma formation. Thereafter, it may be loosely taped to the abdomen.

Ongoing care

1. Formation of the fistula normally takes two to three weeks. During this time, the fixation plate should not be removed. One exception to this rule is if the patient is dehydrated at the time of the gastrostomy insertion. For these patients, the reperfusion of the tissues following administration of fluids will lead to a tightening around the gastrostomy. If the position of the fixation plate is not readjusted to accommodate this, the patient will experience discomfort as ulceration may occur under the fixation plate.
2. Bathing should be avoided unless the fistula has healed.
3. Check site daily for signs of inflammation or exudate.
4. Ensure that the external fixation device is positioned correctly (Box 5.5) and that it has not migrated into the stomach. This can be done by monitoring the length of the tube at the fixation plate.
5. Once healed, the PEG site may be cleaned daily with soft disposable cloths, mild soap and clean water. Cleansing must become part of the patient's daily hygiene. The PEG site must be dried thoroughly following cleansing as moisture will contribute to infection and skin breakdown.
6. When bathing or showering, ensure the PEG end and clamp are closed and that the PEG site is dried thoroughly afterwards.
7. Unless prescribed, avoid the use of creams and talcum powder around the PEG site. Creams may cause the fixation device to slip, leading to tube migration, whilst talcum powder will increase the risk of infection and skin breakdown.
8. No dressing should be necessary around the PEG tube unless there is continued discharge. If discharge is present, the source of the problem should be identified and where possible remedied before dressing the site. For further information on causes of discharge around PEG sites see the ***Complications associated with gastrostomy/jejunostomy feeding tubes*** section below.

Box 5.5 The external fixation plate

The external fixation device, or bolster, is a small piece of polyurethane or silicone. It is usually circular or triangular in shape and encircles the gastrostomy tube. They are designed to anchor the tube externally and to prevent it from being pulled into the stomach.

The external fixation plate is present on PEG, balloon and some radiological gastrostomies. The correct positioning of the external fixation plate is essential to minimise complications.

A loosely secured gastrostomy has the freedom to slide in and out of the tract. This constant movement can lead to the patient having a variety of problems, including:

- erythema (redness) around the PEG site
- inflammation
- feeling of soreness or irritation often extending from the abdomen into the stomach
- exudate or bleeding around or within the fistula
- visible shortening of the available tube outside the abdomen
- overgranulation tissue
- infection

The fixation device should be placed approximately 2–3 mm away from the abdominal skin surface with consideration given to the extension and deflation of the abdomen during breathing, laughing, coughing, sneezing, straining at stool or general position changes. Positioning should be monitored to ensure that once secured the fixation device is neither too tight, increasing the risk of possible tissue necrosis and ulceration, nor too loose, which would allow excessive tube movement in and out of the stomach.

When the tract is established, one method of minimising incorrect positioning is to mark the gastrostomy tube with an indelible marker at the point where the external fixation device should be secured. This may need to be adjusted if the patient gains or loses weight.

9. Advancing and rotating the tube: once the fistula has healed, the PEG tube must be rotated weekly to ensure correct stoma formation, to prevent adherence of the internal bumper to the epithelial lining of the stomach and to prevent overgranulation at the PEG site.

To advance and rotate the PEG tube:
   (i) Release the fixation device.
   (ii) Clean the PEG site and tube thoroughly.
   (iii) Gently push the PEG tube into the abdomen approximately 1–2 cm. There should be no resistance. (If it feels as though

the tube is not moving or is folding into itself, this should be reported to your nutrition nurse specialist, Nutrition Support Team or department that placed the PEG.)

(iv)   Once the PEG has been advanced into the abdomen, rotate the tube 360°. Note that rotation of a PEG tube alone is not sufficient. The internal bumper can still become embedded in the gastric mucosa, even if the tube is rotated on a daily basis. It is the advancing of the internal bumper away from the gastric mucosa (to ensure that it is free) that is important.

(v)   Once the tube has been advanced and rotated, gently pull the tube back out of the abdomen until resistance is felt.

(vi)   Replace the fixation plate.

Radiologically inserted gastrostomy

Care as for the PEG tube, but:

1. Note a RIG tube does not have a clamp. Pinching or bending the tube will shorten its life. Raise the tip of the tube when removing the tip to minimise leakage of gastric contents.
2. Monitor the external length of tube. If the tube appears to have lengthened or there appears to be excess movement in and out of the abdomen but the external fixation plate is correctly positioned, seek assistance. The internal security device may have snapped.

Balloon/button gastrostomy

Care as for PEG, plus:

1. Rotate tube daily. This prevents adhesions to the tract and soreness under the external base.
2. Check and change water in the retention balloon on a weekly basis or as per manufacturer's recommendations (Box 5.6).
3. Monitor for signs of burst balloon (see ***Complications associated with gastrostomy/jejunostomy feeding tubes*** section below).

Aftercare of jejunal feeding tubes

Percutaneous endoscopic gastrojejunostomy

Care as for PEG tube, except:

1. Do not rotate the tube: it may dislodge the jejunal extension. Advance the tube into the abdomen (as per PEG) only. If the

Box 5.6 Changing the water in a balloon or button gastrostomy

---

Balloon gastrostomy

This is best carried out with the patient lying down.

- Have two syringes available – one empty and the second with the required amount of sterile water as stated on the balloon port of the tube.
- Release the external flange and gently push the gastrostomy into the abdomen approximately 2 cm (in most patients this will lead you to the 6 cm marker) to avoid accidentally pulling the tube out whilst the balloon is deflated.
- Attach the empty syringe to the valve port and deflate the balloon by withdrawing the water into the syringe.
- Dispose of first syringe and use the second to insert the required amount of sterile water through the valve port to re-inflate the balloon.
- Once the balloon is re-inflated, remove the syringe and gently pull on the gastrostomy until resistance is felt (i.e. the balloon is inflated).
- Secure the fixation plate in its correct position (approximately 2–3 mm away from the abdominal wall).
- If further verification of tube position is required:
  ○ check tube markers
  ○ withdraw aspirate and measure pH.

If you are feeling resistance or the patient complains of discomfort, you may be trying to inflate the balloon in the tract. Check that you have not accidentally pulled it out from the stomach. Deflate the balloon again and push the tube in further.

However, don't push the tube in too far: this may lead to the tip of the tube passing through the pyloric sphincter. If you inflate the balloon here, the stomach can't empty, as it is obstructed. This will result in abdominal discomfort, vomiting and tube leakage.

Button gastrostomy

As above, but obviously you do not have a flange to release or the comfort of being able to advance the tube into the abdomen.

To prevent accidental removal, keep one hand on the button tube until the balloon is re-inflated.

---

patient starts feeling nauseous, vomits or complains of abdominal discomfort, the position of the tip of the jejunal tube will need to be checked.

2. Ensure regular flushes are given through the jejunal extension to prevent the tube from blocking as they are often only a 9 fr (ch) tube.

3. Do not open the screw connection holding the jejunal tube in place, as it will dislodge the tube.

Surgical jejunostomy

1. Care as for NJ tubes.
2. Unlike gastrostomy tubes, the external fixation plate is not meant to be moved. It may be the only means of securing the tube in the jejunum (see explanation of different jejunal tubes above in the *Surgically placed needle catheter jejunostomy* section).
3. If the device you are caring for has sutures at the abdomen, do not remove them. The sutures will loosen over time as the skin heals. If the sutures are removed, there is a risk of the tube becoming dislodged. Where the jejunostomy is required for long-term feeding, the tube will need to be re-sutured to the abdomen. However, if it is required only for short periods, it is possible to use a security device, such as a StatLock, providing that all those involved in the patient's care are aware that it is the only means of holding the tube in position and any traction or accidental pulling could dislodge the tube completely.
4. If long-term use is required, a better option may be to use a surgical jejunostomy with a Dacron cuff.

Complications associated with gastrostomy/jejunostomy feeding tubes

It is worth noting that most patients experience few problems with their gastrostomy/jejunostomy tubes. However, should your patient have any problems, use the following as a troubleshooting guide to assist you.

Inflammation

Inflammation is a non-specific local reaction to tissue damage or bacterial invasion and is an essential part of the healing process. However, repetitive mechanical trauma caused by movement or pressure from the gastrostomy tube prolongs the inflammatory process. Where inflammation is associated with infection, treatment with systemic antibiotics may be required.

Where a gastrostomy is positioned in a fold of skin at the abdomen and irritation or 'digging in' is a problem, a dry keyhole gauze dressing placed under the fixation device may provide some relief. However, the fixation plate will need to be adjusted to accommodate the dressing and the site cleaned and monitored daily.

Overgranulation

Overgranulation tissue, or granuloma, is formed by a temporary latticework of vascularised connective tissue during the proliferative stage of healing and occurs when the development of granulation tissue during epithelialisation continues after the wound defect has been filled (Myers, 2004). It appears as a raised area extending above the surface of the surrounding epithelium and prevents further healing. Overgranulation tissue will often have high levels of exudate, bleed easily, be painful when touched and provide an ideal environment for bacterial activity.

Inflammation and overgranulation around enteral feeding tubes are essentially preventable problems. The correct positioning of the external fixation device to minimise excessive tube movement on a PEG or the correct fitting of a button tube will minimise the risk of development and limit the need for medical intervention.

A number of dressings are used in the treatment of overgranulation tissue, with varying success, including:

- **Foam dressings (e.g. Lyofoam or Biatin):** The application of foam dressing applied directly onto the affected tissue to suppress the overgranulation tissue is often used as a first line of treatment. The fixation plate or shaft length will need to be adjusted to accommodate the extra padding. Use of these dressings for up to five days should suppress growth. For smaller areas of overgranulation, one layer of foam is often sufficient, but for larger areas a double layer of foam may be required for at least one week before changing to a single layer.
- **Silver nitrate sticks** were previously a very popular means of burning overgranulation tissue. Unfortunately, their application can be quite uncomfortable for the patient. It causes a stinging and throbbing sensation which persists for some time after application, and unless the underlying problem is treated overgranulation tissue grows back.
- **Silver dressings:** There are a number of silver dressings available (e.g. Actisorb Silver 220 or Contreet) which have been found useful (Leak, 2002). They have the benefit of not only diminishing overgranulation tissue but also reducing the colonisation of bacteria.

- **Steroid cream** applied directly onto the overgranulation tissue is usually effective – just avoid contact with the feeding tube. This method of treatment should only be used for short periods (i.e. no longer than seven days)
- **Systemic antibiotics:** Where infection is present, a course of systemic antibiotics may be required. Treatment with topical antibiotics is not normally recommended.

If these interventions are not effective, the enteral feeding tube may be replaced with either a smaller gauge tube or it may require re-siting. However, these measures should not be used as the first line of management.

Breakages to external adaptors

It is not unusual for the ends of feeding tubes to become worn and damaged through wear and tear. If the tube in need of repair is a PEG or RIG, the ends can be easily replaced. However, if the ends of a balloon gastrostomy/jejunostomy is in situ, the whole tube will need replacing.

Burst balloon

The balloon should be deflated and re-inflated with the required amount of sterile water once a week or as per manufacturer's recommendations.

If there appears to be excessive movement of the gastrostomy in and out of the stoma or more than 10% of the balloon volume has been lost over the previous week, the balloon may have burst. If so, the tube will need to be replaced.

Problems that may cause a balloon to burst include:

- overfilled balloon, making its structure weaker
- fungal infection: if the fungal infection is not treated before changing the tube, the infection will simply transfer to the new tube
- incorrect shaft length (too short) in a button gastrostomy, causing pressure on the balloon
- gastric pH, particularly a very acid environment
- medication.

Leakage around the stoma/fistula site

Leakage may occur if the internal bolster or balloon is not correctly positioned.

Check that:

- there is resistance on the tube when gently pulled at the abdomen
- tube markings are as recorded
- tube length has not shortened
- the correct size tube has been fitted.

Tube blockages

Some of the most common causes of enteral feeding tube blockages include:

- failure to flush the tube at regular intervals
- administration of partially crushed medication
- feed/drug interaction.

Before running for the syringe to release the blockage, it is also worth checking that the patient is not sitting or lying on their tube, that it has not kinked or become twisted or that the clamp is closed.

Preventing a tube blockage is in the interests of the patient and the nurse. Attempting to unblock an enteral feeding tube is often time-consuming and, unless addressed promptly, may prove unsuccessful, particularly with nasogastric or NJ tubes. Failure to relieve the blockage may mean having to replace the blocked tube, causing unnecessary stress and discomfort to the patient and a further delay in feeding.

Historically a number of methods have been used to unblock enteral feeding tubes with varying degrees of success, including:

- warm water
- soda water
- flat carbonated drinks, such as lemonade or cola
- pineapple juice
- pancreatic enzymes.

Studies have shown that water is as effective as any other solution in unblocking enteral feeding tubes (Metheny, 1988).

Cola not only stains the tube but also the acid environment it creates may exacerbate the blockage and damage the fabric of the tube. Pancreatic enzymes are effective but expensive.

However, flushing may not be the first action to take when attempting to unblock an enteral feeding tube. Once you have checked that the tube is not kinked or the patient lying on it, try rolling the tube gently between the forefinger and thumb to breakdown or dislodge the blockage. Attempts should then be made to aspirate as much of the tube contents back up the tube into a syringe. Only then should any fluid be inserted into the tube. If medication is the cause of the blockage, pushing the build up into the stomach may cause the patient harm.

(NB: Under no circumstances should excessive force or sharp instruments be used to resolve a blockage.)

Knotting of jejunal extension tubes

This is a risk with a jejunal extension tube fed through a PEG (i.e. a PEGJ tube). The tip of the jejunal extension may become dislodged as the endoscope is removed, during the insertion procedure, or, if too long a length of tubing is inserted through the PEG (in the hope that it will spontaneously pass through into the small intestine), retrograde movement of the tube into the stomach may occur. It is important only to insert the required length of tube for that individual patient. Once the tube has knotted, it is difficult to resolve.

Feed-related issues

Diarrhoea

In the majority of cases, the cause of diarrhoea is not related to the feed but to the patient's medical condition. If a case of diarrhoea persists, a stool specimen should be taken to exclude gastrointestinal infection.

Other possible causes of diarrhoea to consider include:

- Medication side effects: is the patient taking a course of antibiotics or have they just completed a course? Are they receiving a number of liquid preparations (see **Drug administration through an enteral feeding tube** section below)? Discuss options with the pharmacist or doctor.
- Is the feed being administered too quickly? Reducing the rate by 10–20 ml/hr may reduce the incidence of diarrhoea. Discuss this option with the patient's dietitian.
- The feed being administered is too cold. This may be more of a problem for patients being cared for in their own home where boxes of feed are stored in a garage over the winter period. Enteral feed should be administered at room temperature. Where stored

in a cold environment, the feed should be allowed to warm to room temperature before being used.

- Bacterial contamination of feed and/or equipment. This is rarely a problem as all readily prepared feeds and giving sets are sterile. Check handling procedures. If a problem is suspected with the feed, seal the container, label it and send it to microbiology. Do not leave enteral feed hanging for over 24 hours.
- Lack of fibre: discuss with the dietitian.

Constipation

Possible causes of constipation include:

- medication, e.g. opiates
- dehydration: ensure that sufficient fluid is being taken. Check regimen to ensure all feed and water flushes are being given. Give additional flushes of water if fluid requirements increase, e.g. in hot weather or the patient develops a pyrexia
- lack of dietary fibre
- medical condition: liaise with medical staff
- reduced mobility
- please note that the patient may require regular aperients in order to prevent constipation.

Nausea/abdominal distension

Possible causes of nausea or abdominal distension include:

- the feed is being administered too quickly: consider reducing the rate of feeding (discuss this with the ward dietitian)
- patient being fed whilst lying flat: adjust the patient to ensure they are propped up to at least a 35° angle
- a too rapid administration of feed using the bolus method; discuss with the patient's dietitian reducing the amount of feed administered per bolus or the rate at which it is given.

Gastrostomy removal

Planned removal

Where removal is as a result of the patient managing to meet their nutritional requirements orally, it is advisable to ensure the patient is able to maintain their weight for a minimum period of one month without using the enteral feeding tube for nutrition prior to it being removed.

If a **PEG** is in situ, removal is either endoscopic or performed by cutting the tube close to the abdomen and allowing the internal button/bolster to pass spontaneously through the gastrointestinal tract. Whilst this method is quicker, easier and more cost-effective to perform than an endoscopy, there is always a risk that the bolster may not pass spontaneously. Therefore, the patient must be carefully assessed by the gastroenterologist, nutrition nurse specialist or Nutrition Support Team before a PEG tube is removed using this method.

Some PEGs are devised to be traction-removable. Although this sounds a far better option with the PEG being removed at the patient's bedside, in reality these tubes are often very difficult to remove and may require intravenous sedation or endoscopic removal.

A **RIG** is removed by releasing or cutting the cotton string which allows the 'pigtail' in the abdomen to unravel. Once the 'pigtail' is released, the tube can be removed percutaneously by pulling it out through the abdomen.

A **balloon** or **button gastrostomy** is removed by deflating the balloon and, with gentle traction, pull the tube out of the abdomen.

Depending upon the type of **surgical jejunostomy** in place, removal may be via traction or a surgical cutdown procedure.

Accidental tube removal

Under normal circumstances it is rare for a PEG tube to fall out. There is a slightly higher risk with a radiological, balloon or button gastrostomy.

If a gastrostomy or jejunostomy is removed within the weeks of a primary intubation, the tract will not be fully formed. There is a risk that any tube inserted percutaneously will not safely reach the stomach but may become incorrectly positioned in the peritoneal cavity, putting the patient at risk of developing peritonitis. Therefore, if the feeding tube has been in place for less than three weeks, do not attempt to insert a tube percutaneously. Cover the site with a sterile dressing, commence prophylactic IV antibiotics and seek to provide another method of nutrition support, for example nasogastric feeding until the old stoma site has healed and/or advice has been sought from the team that places the relevant feeding tube in your area.

If the gastrostomy tube has been in place for over three weeks, a balloon or button gastrostomy can be inserted percutaneously.

If no attempt is made to pass a tube, the tract will start to close within a couple of hours, making a percutaneous replacement of a feeding tube difficult. The stoma normally closes completely within eight to 24 hours. If the stoma closes, a new feeding tube will need to be sited.

If there are no further plans to use the tract for enteral tube feeding, the remaining fistula should be covered with a sterile permeable dressing for at least 24 hours.

Enteral tube feeds

There are many different enteral tube feeds available; check which ones are commonly used in your area, as they are made by different companies.

In general terms, the feeds fall into broad categories, which may vary slightly in composition and amount of electrolytes.

Osmolality

Osmolality is the number of osmotically active particles in a kilogram of solvent. The osmolality of plasma is normally 280–300 mOsmol/kg, and the body attempts to keep the osmolality of the contents of the stomach and intestine at an isotonic level. This is by producing intestinal secretions, which dilute a concentrated meal or drink. If an enteral feed with a high osmolality is administered, intestinal secretions can rapidly be produced in large quantities to effectively reduce the osmolality – potentially causing diarrhoea.

Therefore, in order to avoid diarrhoea, high osmolality feeds should be administered slowly.

Common enteral feeds

These are generally presented in ready-to-use sterile containers, although exact presentation varies between companies.

Most standard feeds can hang for 24 hours, after which time any remaining feed should be discarded.

The standard feeds are whole-protein (polymeric), and therefore require an intact gut to enable their digestion and absorption.

Standard feeds

These are 1 kcal/ml feeds, and are often used as an initial feed or when needing to ensure adequate fluid intake without needing additional water.

- Osmolality: 288–315 mOsmol/kg H_2O
- These types of feeds are usually nutritionally complete in 1500 ml/1500 kcal.
- Examples include: Fresubin Original, Nutrison Standard, Osmolite, Ensure, Isosource Standard.
- Common volumes available: 500 ml, 1000 ml, 1500 ml

Fibre feed

These again are 1 kcal/ml and are often used when long-term feeding is required, or if constipation or diarrhoea is a problem.

- Osmolality: 250–300 mOsmol/kg H_2O
- Usually nutritionally complete in 1500 ml/1500 kcal
- Examples include: Nutrison Multifibre, Jevity, Fresubin Original Fibre, Isosource Fibre, Novasource GI Control
- Common volumes available: 500 ml, 1000 ml, 1500 ml

High-energy feed

These are 1.2–1.6 kcal/ml, not usually used as a first feed, but once feeding is established useful to cut down volume and consequently time spent feeding, also useful for overnight feeding once established in order to maximise energy in small volume. Useful if patients have high-nutrition requirements, for example burns, Huntington's chorea, or low-fluid requirements or fluid restriction.

- Osmolality: 359–510 mOsmol/kg H_2O
- Usually nutritionally complete in 1500 kcal/1000 ml
- Examples include: Fresubin Energy, Nutrison Energy, Ensure Plus, Isosource Energy, Osmolite Plus
- Common volumes available: 500 ml, 1000 ml, 1500 ml

High-energy fibre feed

As above, 1.2–1.5 kcal/ml; again, useful for long-term feeding to help normalise bowel movements.

- Osmolality: 420–524 mOsmol/kg H_2O
- Usually nutritionally complete in 1500 kcal/1000 ml
- Examples include: Nutrison Energy Multifibre, Fresubin Energy Fibre, Isosource Energy Fibre, Jevity 1.5 kcal, Jevity Plus, Novasource Forte
- Common volumes available: 500 ml, 1000 ml, 1500 ml

Low-energy nutritionally complete feeds

Some feeds are nutritionally complete at lower energy levels. They tend to have higher protein and electrolyte content, tend to contain fibre and tend to be used long term. They are useful for long-term feeding in people with low-nutritional requirements, for example in multiple sclerosis (MS), motor neurone disease (MND), bed bound following stroke (CVA) etc.

- Osmolality: 250–420 mOsmol/kg H_2O
- Examples include: Nutrison 1000 Complete Multifibre, Fresubin 1000 Complete, Nutrison 1200 Complete Multifibre, Fresubin 1200 Complete
- Usually nutritionally complete in 1000–1200 kcal
- Common volume available: 1000 ml

Specialised enteral feeds

Low-sodium feed

This is a specific feed for use when strict sodium restriction is required, for example in liver patients with ascites. Other constituents of this type of feed are similar to standard feeds.

- Osmolality: 240 mOsmol/kg H_2O
- Nutritionally complete in 1500 ml/1500 kcal
- Example: Nutrison Low Sodium
- Common volumes available: 500 ml, 1000 ml

High-protein feed

With or without fibre.

- Osmolality: 355–425 mOsmol/kg H_2O
- Examples include: Fresubin HP Energy, Nutrison Protein Plus, Nutrison Protein Plus Multifibre, Perative, Jevity Promote
- Common volume available: 100 ml

Soya feed

This is for patients intolerant to cow's milk protein.

- Osmolality: 295 mOsmol/kg H_2O
- Example: Nutrison Soya

Soya feed with fibre
This is also for patients intolerant to cow's milk protein.

- Osmolality: 275 mOsmol/kg H_2O
- Example: Nutrison Soya Multifibre

Disease-specific feeds

There are a number of disease-specific feeds available, including:

- **Renal feeds:** concentrated/low-electrolyte feeds suitable for fluid restriction
- **Gastrointestinal feeds:** 'pre-digested' elemental/peptide feeds, consisting of basic nutritional building blocks, such as amino acids or peptides (rather than whole-protein), and simple fat and carbohydrates
- **Respiratory feeds:** contain higher proportion of fat, which produces less carbon dioxide when metabolised
- **Cancer feed:** contains eicosapentaenoic acid (EPA) to help prevent cancer cachexia
- **Immune feeds:** containing additional specific amino acids or fats
- **Diabetic feeds:** there has been discussion regarding specific feeds for diabetics; although there are some feeds in use in Europe, they are not yet in use in the United Kingdom.

In practice, most patients' needs will be met by one or a combination of the above feeds. This is the safest way of ensuring a patient receives nutrition, as the pre-packaged feeds, if handled correctly, offer the smallest chance of becoming contaminated.

Feed contamination

To reduce the risk of microbial contamination, pre-prepared sterile enteral feeds should not hang for more than 24 hours (Clinical Resource Efficiency Support Team, 2004). Once a sterile feed has been opened, it must be used within 24 hours or discarded. If a sterile feed that requires decanting into a sterile reservoir is being used, a strict aseptic technique must be performed and the feed should be discarded after 24 hours.

In some specialist units, feeds may be made up from modular-type ingredients – adding separate fat, carbohydrate and protein modules. These feeds are more flexible, but there is a greater risk of contamination, and the feed cannot hang for as long on a warm ward. A maximum of four hours is the recommended hanging time for non-sterile feeds (Payne-James *et al.*, 1992).

Feed administration

Feeding should only be commenced once the position of the enteral feeding tube has been confirmed and usually in conjunction with a feeding regimen following an assessment by the dietitian of nutritional needs. The delivery of feed may be via continuous infusion using a pump, intermittent infusion (with or without a pump) or bolus feeding. The method of administration used will depend upon the patient's ability to tolerate the feed, their medical acuity, nutritional requirements and preferences. The feed should be stored and administered at room temperature. Administering feed which has been stored in a refrigerator can cause gastric discomfort. During feeding and for at least an hour after feeding stops, the patient should be positioned with their head and shoulders raised to an angle of approximately 30° and be monitored closely for any potential side effects (as discussed above).

When the decision is made that nutritional support is no longer necessary, there is usually a phased reduction with continued monitoring, to ensure that the patient can continue to maintain their nutritional status without support. This may mean a reduction in the volume of enteral feeding, or oral supplements or snacks received, whilst weight and overall dietary intake are still being monitored. In the same way that nutritional care is escalated using a step-by-step approach, it is good practice to reduce it using the same approach.

Pumps

Where a continuous administration of feed is necessary, a feeding pump specifically designed for use with enteral feeding systems should be used. Most companies produce their own pump designed to fit their own giving sets. Pumps designed for IV administration should not be used (Department of Health, 2004). The type of pump used will vary upon the patient's level of activity. Larger pumps tend to be used in hospital, but upon discharge there is often the option to supply the patient with a smaller ambulatory pump, which can be fitted into a rucksack to be carried on the patient's back or onto a wheelchair, providing some level of freedom whilst the feed is administered.

Box 5.7   Alternative formulations

- Liquid medication
- Dispersible tablets
- Suppositories
- Transdermal patches
- Injection (unlicensed)

Drug administration through an enteral feeding tube

Legal implications of crushing tablets

Crushing tablets, opening capsules and administration via feeding tubes generally fall outside a drug's product licence. Where a preparation is altered and the patient has an adverse reaction, liability does not lie with the pharmaceutical company but with the healthcare professional involved in the drug's provision and administration (British Association for Parenteral and Enteral Nutrition, 2003).

The alteration of a formulation to aid compliance or to administer medication via a feeding tube is common practice. However, crushing the tablets or opening capsules contrary to the prescribing practitioner would be in breach of the Medicines Act 1968 (James, 2004). It is therefore essential that if tablets need to be crushed the nurse seeks advice from a pharmacist before administration.

In most cases, alternative products can be sourced that would make this practice unnecessary (Box 5.7). Pharmacists should be contacted before or very soon after the insertion of an enteral feeding tube for a thorough review of medication and to check the availability of alternative formulations. For example, a patient prescribed isosorbide mononitrate tablets could be switched to a GTN transdermal patch to avoid the need for crushing tablets.

Clinical implications of altering a formulation

Medicines are available in a number of formulations, including sustained release (SR) or modified release (MR). It is essential these are swallowed whole. If an MR preparation were crushed, the drug would be released in one 'hit' rather than the intended duration of action of 12–24 hours. This results in the patient receiving an immediate overdose followed by an extended period without medication. It is for this reason that SR or MR preparations should not be altered, i.e. crushed or opened (Morris, 2005).

Enteric-coated drugs bypass the stomach and are released further down in the intestine. The aim of this is to either reduce irritation caused by the release of the drug in the stomach, for example non-steroidal anti-inflammatory drugs (NSAIDs), or to deliver the drug to a more appropriate site of action. If the enteric coating is destroyed by crushing the tablet, the drug will be released directly in the stomach.

Cytotoxic, hormone, immunosuppressant and steroid medication should not be crushed, because of the health risk to the nurse whilst crushing the medication, as airborne particles of the drug may be inhaled.

Liquid medications are the preferred formulation for administration via an enteral feeding tube. However, where a patient receives a number of sugar-free liquid preparations, the total sorbitol content of the medicines administered should be considered. Sorbitol or other artificial sweeteners may cause flatulence or diarrhoea (particularly if the tip of the tube sits in the jejunum). Diarrhoea will in turn affect the level of drug absorbed by the patient. Therefore, this could have implications for the patient receiving four or five liquid preparations.

Problems encountered when administering drugs via enteral feeding tubes

Coagulation of the drug and the feed

This is commonly caused by acidic mixtures, for example chlorpheniramine, promethazine, thioridazine or antacids containing aluminium, calcium or magnesium coming into contact with the feed. Water flushes must be given before and on completion of the administration of the medications.

Reduced drug absorption

Feed can reduce the absorption of phenytoin, ciprofloxacin, theophylline, and warfarin. It could also affect drugs which need to be given on an empty stomach for maximum absorption, for example penicillin, flucloxacillin, ketoconazole and tetracyclines. If possible, these drugs should be given once daily to minimise the interruption of feeding times. The feed should be **stopped two hours before administration** and the tube flushed with water, then restarted two hours after the drug has been given. In some clinical situations, larger doses may be required to compensate for reduced absorption.

Drug binding with the tube

To minimise this problem (for example when using phenytoin, carbamazepine), it is essential that the enteral feeding tube is flushed thoroughly following the administration of these drugs. Using a 'push pause' method of fluid administration may also reduce adherence to the internal lumen.

Crushed tablets blocking the tube if not finely powdered

If there is a liquid preparation or soluble tablet available, then these are the preferred first-line preparations for enteral tube feeding.

Coagulation of granules

The contents of capsules (granules), when wet, can cause blockage. This commonly occurs with enteric-coated granules, for example omeprazole (highly acid labile). If it is essential that this preparation be used, the contents of the capsule should be placed into a dry medicine pot and only six to 10 granules administered at a time, flushed with 10–20 ml of water. Alternatively, omeprazole granules may be dissolved in 10–20 ml sodium bicarbonate 8.4%. However, owing to the likelihood of tube blockage, the use of lansoprazole dispersible tablets is a better option for administration through an enteral feeding tube.

How to give medicines via the enteral feeding tube

If tablets must be crushed or the contents of capsules used, this should be done in a pestle and mortar and the powder mixed with plenty of water. Some compressed tablets can be dissolved by placing inside a dry syringe (by removing the plunger), adding a small amount of water and leaving to dissolve. Thicker liquid preparations may require dilution to ensure the patient receives the required dose and to minimise the risk of blockages.

Each medicine should be administered separately to minimise interactions between drugs and/or feed. Medication should not be administered while the enteral feed is in progress. If a feed is in progress, it should be stopped and the enteral feeding tube flushed with at least 30 ml of water. Medication can then be given. The tube should be flushed with at least 10 ml of water between medications to ensure each drug has been cleared from the tube. The size of the flush given may vary, depending upon the number of medications given and the patient's fluid requirements. The tube should be flushed with at least 30 ml of water following the administration of the last drug (British Association for Parenteral and Enteral Nutrition, 2003).

The preferred method of administration of medication is in liquid form or, where that is not possible, a dispersible preparation. It should be noted, however, that dispersible tablets should be dissolved in plenty of water as small amounts of undissolved tablet may block an enteral feeding tube, especially where the flushing technique is poor or infrequent. Regular administration of medications and a lack of flushing can cause of build-up of residue on the inner lumen of the feeding tube, making it more likely to block.

Nurses should be aware of the position of the tip of the nasogastric tube before administering medication. If the tip has progressed into the small intestine, absorption of some drugs may be affected, for example digoxin, as it is primarily absorbed in the stomach.

Syringe use

Using intravenous syringes to measure and administer oral medicines through enteral feeding tubes has unfortunately led to a number of fatalities through the inadvertent administration of oral medications into intravenous access. In response to these incidents, the National Patient Safety Agency (NPSA) released an alert: *Promoting safer measurement and administration of liquid medicines via oral and other enteral routes* (2007); see Box 5.8. In this alert, the NPSA states that specifically designed enteral syringes must be used for:

- the measuring of oral liquid medication to be given orally.
- the measurement and administration of oral medication through all enteral feeding tubes.

Box 5.8   Enteral routes

The enteral route includes:

- oral
- via nasogastric or NJ tubes
- via PEGs or PEGJs
- rectal

The term 'oral liquid medicine' refers to:

- soluble tablets once dissolved, e.g. paracetamol
- liquid preparations, e.g. Oramorph, baclofen
- enteral feeds
- flushes (include water, sodium chloride 0.9% and air).

These syringes should be purple in colour and clearly labelled 'for oral/enteral use'.

Oral syringes are designed with a wider neck that makes them incompatible with all IV equipment. However, using an oral syringe to administer medication through an enteral feeding tube requires an adaptor, which makes the syringe compatible with IV equipment once more. Their use is therefore not recommended for this purpose.

The only time an IV syringe should be used with an enteral feeding tube is to inflate the retention balloon of a low-profile device, as the valve will only connect to an IV syringe (National Patient Safety Agency, 2007).

Further information

The British Association for Parenteral and Enteral Nutrition (BAPEN; 2003) has published posters and information booklets for nurses, patients and GPs to clarify issues surrounding the safe administration of medication through enteral tubes. These can be obtained from the BAPEN website at: www.bapen.org.uk/res_drugs.html.

Flushing enteral feeding tubes

The flushing of any enteral feeding tube with water is essential to help the patient meet their fluid requirements and decrease the risk of tube blockage or microbial contamination.

An enteral feeding tube should be flushed:

- before a feed is commenced and on its completion
- before, between and after administration of each individual medication
- if the patient is disconnected from the feed.

If the patient is not using their tube to regularly receive enteral feed or fluid, the tube should be flushed with 30–50 ml of water once or twice daily to maintain tube patency.

The type of water used for flushing enteral feeding tubes is dependent upon local hospital policy. The general rule is that for patients who are *not* immunocompromised cooled boiled water or freshly run water taken from a drinking source can be used. For patients who *are* immunocompromised, sterile water must be used. Sterile water is also required for patients being fed into the small intestine.

It is preferable that a larger, 50 ml, syringe be used to flush. Smaller syringes will not only require more time and effort in having to refill the syringe but also repeated use creates additional pressure within the tube, which may cause splitting in a weakened tube.

There are two methods in which water flushes are commonly given:

- bolus (using the plunger)
- gravity (with the plunger removed).

The gravity method is useful if large amounts of water have to be administered at one time. Unfortunately, it does not provide the turbulence required within the feeding tube to remove any build-up of feed or medication that will occur in the inner lumen of the feeding tube over time. Bolus administration will provide the turbulence required and help prevent the occurrence of tube blockages but can be more time-consuming if large volumes of fluid are required. The patient should receive water flushes using bolus administration at least once a day. When using the bolus method, further turbulence can be created by using a 'push pause' technique. Using this method causes the water flush to move in all directions within the tube and therefore be more effective at dislodging particles of feed or medication.

Conclusion

The need for some level of enteral nutrition support is common within all hospitals in the United Kingdom. Using a step-by-step approach generally provides a safe means of administration. However, there are still risks attached with each level of nutrition support, and nursing staff must be able to recognise the risks and the actions required to minimise them. Before commencing nutrition support, consideration will also need to be given to the most appropriate method of feed administration, balancing issues around what actions are in the patient's best interests, the likely outcome of therapy and the patient's preference.

References

Allison, S.P. (1999) *Hospital Food as Treatment: A report by a working party of the British Association for Parenteral and Enteral Nutrition*, BAPEN, Maidenhead.
Anderson, M., O'Connor, M., Mayer, P. *et al.* (2004) The nasal loop provides an alternative to percutaneous endoscopic gastrostomy in high-risk dysphagic stroke patients. *Clinical Nutrition* **23** (4), 501–6.
Bowling, T. (2004) *Nutritional Support for Adults and Children: A handbook for hospital practice*, Radcliffe Medical Press, Abingdon.
British Association for Parenteral and Enteral Nutrition (2003) Administering drugs via enteral feeding tubes: A practical guide, www.bapen.org.uk, accessed 24 June 2007.
Burnham, P. (2000) A guide to nasogastric tube intubation. *Nursing Times* (Nutrition Supplement) **96** (8), S6–7.
Cannaby, A., Evans, L., Freeman, A. (2002) Nursing care of patients with a nasogastric tube. *British Journal of Nursing* **11** (6), 366–72.
Clinical Resource Efficiency Support Team (2004) *Guidelines for the Management of Enteral Tube Feeding in Adults*, CREST, Central Medical Advisory Committee, Northern Ireland.
Colagiovanni, L. (1999) Taking the tube. *Nursing Times* **95** (21), 63–7.
Davies, A.R., Froomes, P.R.A., French, C.J. *et al.* (2002) Randomised comparison of nasojejunal and nasogastric feeding in critically ill patients. *Critical Care Medicine* **30** (3), 586–90.
Department of Health (2000) *Better Hospital Food: The NHS Plan*, DH, London.
Department of Health (2001) *Essence of Care: Patient-focused benchmarking for healthcare practitioners*, DH, London.
Department of Health (2004) *Building a Safer NHS for Patients: Improving medication safety: A report by the Chief Pharmaceutical Officer*, DH, London.
Department of Health (2007) *Improving Nutritional Care: A joint action plan from the Department of Health and Nutrition Summit stakeholders*, DH, London.
Dewar, H. (1997) Nasogastric tube audit: standard setting and review of specifications. *Journal of Human Nutrition and Dietetics* **10**, 313–15.
Dougherty, L., Lister, S. (2008) *The Royal Marsden Hospital Manual of Clinical Nursing Procedures*, 7th edn, Blackwell Publishing, Oxford.
Elia, M. (1996) Special nutritional problems and the use of enteral and parenteral nutrition, in *Oxford Textbook of Medicine* (eds D.J. Weatherall, J.G.G. Ledingham, D.A. Warrell), Oxford Medical Publications, Oxford.
Elia, M., Stratton, R., Russell, C. *et al.* (2005) *The cost of disease-related malnutrition in the UK and economic considerations for the use of oral nutritional supple-*

ments (ONS) in adults, Health Economics Working Group, British Association for Parenteral and Enteral Nutrition, Maidenhead.

James, A. (2004) The legal and clinical implications of crushing tablet medications. *Nursing Times* **100** (50), 28–9.

Khair, J. (2005) Guidelines for testing the placing of nasogastric tubes. *Nursing Times* **101** (20), 26–7.

Leak, K. (2002) PEG site infections: A novel use for Actisorb Silver 220. *British Journal of Community Nursing* **7** (6), 321–5.

Mahan, L.K., Arlin, M.T. (1992) *Krause's Food, Nutrition & Diet Therapy,* W.B. Saunders & Company, Philadelphia.

Martyn, C.N. (1998) Effect of nutritional status on the use of health care resources by patients with chronic disease living in the community. *Clinical Nutrition* **17** (3), 119–23.

Medicines and Healthcare products Regulatory Agency (2004) Medical Device Alert Ref: MDA 2004/ 026, Enteral Feeding Tubes (nasogastric).

Metheny, N. (1988) Effect of feeding tube properties and three irrigants on clogging rates. *Nursing Research* **37**, 165–9.

Metheny, N., Meert, K.L. (2004) Monitoring feeding tube placement. *Nutrition in Clinical Practice* **19**, 487–95.

Metheny, N., Spies M., Eisenberg, P. (1986) Frequency of nasoenteral tube displacement and associated risk factors. *Research in Nursing and Health* **9** (3), 241–7.

Metheny, N., McSweeny, M., Wehrle, M., Wiersema, L. (1990) Effectiveness of the auscultatory method in predicting feeding tube location. *Nursing Research* **39** (5), 262–6.

Metheny, N., Reed, L., Wiersema, L. (1993) Effectiveness of pH measurements in predicting feeding tube placement: An update. *Nursing Research* **4** (6), 324–31.

Metheny, N.A., Clouse, R.E., Clark, J.M. *et al.* (1994) pH testing of feeding tube aspirates to determine placement. *Nutrition in Clinical Practice* **9**, 185–90.

Morris, H. (2005) Administering drugs to patients with swallowing difficulties. *Nursing Times* **101** (39), 28–30.

Myers, B.A. (2004) Wound healing, in *Wound Management: Principles and Practice,* 2nd edn (ed. B. Myers), Prentice Hall, Upper Saddle River, NJ.

National Institute for Health and Clinical Excellence (2006) *Nutrition Support in Adults: Oral nutrition support, enteral tube feeding and parenteral nutrition, Clinical Guideline 32,* NICE, London.

National Nurses Nutrition Group (2004) Guidelines for confirming correct positioning of nasogastric feeding tubes. Interim guidelines in response to the MRHA (MDA /2004/026) safety alert.

National Patient Safety Agency (2005) *Patient Safety Alert 05: Reducing the harm caused by misplaced nasogastric tubes,* February 21, NPSA, London.

National Patient Safety Agency (2007) *Promoting safer measurement and administration of liquid medicines via oral and other enteral routes,* Ref: NPSA/2007/19 March 2007, NPSA, London.

Payne-James, J.J., Bray, J., Rana, S. *et al.* (1992) Retrograde contamination of enteral feeding delivery systems. *Journal of Parenteral and Enteral Nutrition* **16** (4), 369–73.

Popovich, M.J., Lockrem, J.D., Zivot, J.B. (1996) Nasal bridle revisited: An improvement in the technique to prevent unintentional removal of small nasoenteric feeding tubes. *Critical Care Medicine* **24**, 429–31.

Rollins, H. (1997) A nose for trouble. *Nursing Times* **93** (49), 66–7.

Soulsby, C., Weekes, L. (2004) Estimating nutritional requirements for adults, in *A Pocket Guide to Clinical Nutrition 2004*, (eds. V. Todovoric, A. Micklewright), British Dietetic Association, London.

World Health Organization (2002) *Keep Fit for Life: Meeting the needs of older persons*, WHO, Geneva.

Chapter 6

Parenteral Nutrition

Carolyn Best, Helen Hitchings, Joanna Boult and Harriet Gordon

Introduction

'Parenteral nutrition' (PN) refers to the administration of nutrients via the intravenous (IV) or parenteral route and is widely used to treat or prevent malnutrition both in hospitals and increasingly in the home environment. It is therefore surprising that there is little information regarding current in-patient PN practice in the United Kingdom (Hearnshaw & Thompson, 2007).

In 2006, the National Institute for Health and Clinical Excellence (NICE) published guidelines on nutritional support in adults. The only national guidelines in the United Kingdom regarding PN prior to this were the British Association for Parenteral and Enteral Nutrition (BAPEN) guidelines, dating back to 1996 (Pennington *et al.*, 1996); so it is unsurprising to find differences in practice throughout the country.

It is fairly common to hear the term 'TPN', or total parenteral nutrition, used when discussing the administration of nutrients via the intravenous route. TPN means that the patient receives all their nutritional requirements via the intravenous route. However, as not all patients will receive their total nutritional requirements via this route, it is more appropriate to refer to the administration of intravenous nutrition as 'PN', or parenteral nutrition.

The provision of nutritional support is indicated when nutritional needs cannot be met via the oral route. PN is indicated when the gut is not functional, cannot be accessed or a patient's total nutritional requirements cannot be met by enteral feeding alone (Russell *et al.*, 2002). It should also be considered when starvation occurs, or is likely to occur, for seven or more days (National Institute for Health and Clinical Excellence, 2006).

However, it must be recognised that the provision of PN carries potentially life-threatening risks, as nutrients will be administered directly into the central circulation via a central catheter and therefore should not be started without a proper consideration of both risks and benefits (Pennington, 1990). Where possible, enteral access should be used as it generally carries a lower level of risk. Therefore, before PN is commenced, all options for administration of enteral nutrition should be fully discussed. An unwillingness to eat or a general poor nutritional state is not an indication for PN.

The NICE guidelines (2006) state that PN should be reserved for those patients with a non-functioning, inaccessible or perforated intestine, i.e. where enteral feeding is not possible. Patients should be malnourished (body mass index <18.5 kg m^{-2}) and with unintentional weight loss for three to six months; or be at risk of malnutrition having eaten very little for more than five days and be unlikely to eat more than very small amounts for the next five days.

The guidelines do not list specific conditions that patients referred for PN should present with, but do list characteristics patients may demonstrate to indicate the need for considering PN.

For example:

- signs of gastrointestinal obstruction
- ileus
- dysmotility
- fistulae
- severe malabsorption (to a degree that prevents ample gastrointestinal absorption of nutrients)
- surgical resection.

BAPEN guidelines state that short-term PN may be indicated in patients with mucositis from recent chemotherapy, severe pancreatitis, inflammatory bowel disease (a minority of patients) and multiple-organ failure (Pennington *et al.*, 1996).

There has been a widespread clinical belief that PN in normal clinical use is of little benefit unless it is given for more than seven days. This conclusion was possibly reached following publication of Veterans Affairs Total Parenteral Nutrition Cooperative Study Group (1991), which, when looking at the duration of PN, could only show beneficial effects in malnourished patients fed for seven days or more. However, NICE guidance (2006) states that patients with a definite clinical indication for PN support often demonstrate rapid resolution of the intestinal failure that originally led to them requiring PN (as nutrient deficiencies and adverse changes in metabolism and physiology are rectified). They do not, however, state a recommended minimum duration for PN.

In clinical practice, the majority of PN usage tends to be short-term use (i.e. up to seven days) for in-patients on surgical and intensive/high-dependency care wards. There are, however, a small group of patients that require long-term PN, often needing it to be provided at home. Home PN is only provided from a few specialist centres throughout the United Kingdom.

In patients whose blood levels are stable, it can sometimes be easier to meet their nutritional requirements with PN, as they are not prone to the gastrointestinal complications associated with enteral feeding. It can therefore be easier to increase the level of nutrition provided as it is not reliant on gastrointestinal tolerance.

Indications of parenteral nutrition

- following bowel surgery where the gut will not be functional in the early post-operative phase
- severe inflammatory bowel disease
- severe pancreatitis
- severe mucositis in those undergoing chemotherapy
- multiple-organ failure
- patients whose nutritional requirements cannot be met enterally.

Long-term PN is usually required following:

- intestinal failure (Pennington *et al.*, 1996)
- short bowel syndrome. (This is usually defined by the remaining small intestine measuring less than 200 cm following extensive bowel resection.) If there is 100 cm or more of large bowel remaining, then long-term PN may not be needed as the large bowel will eventually adapt to accommodate enteral feeding
- inflammatory bowel disease, often Crohn's
- intestinal atresia
- radiation enteritis
- motility disorders (e.g. scleroderma, and chronic idiopathic intestinal pseudo-obstruction syndrome).

PN is not indicated:

- when patients can absorb adequate nutrition via the oral route or through enteral tube feeding (Hamilton, 2000)

- when a clear goal of PN cannot be defined
- if it is prolonging life in terminal illness.

Clinical assessment of the patient requiring parenteral nutrition

PN should only be commenced following careful and thorough patient assessment. Patients who have received little or no nutrition for a number of days are at risk of developing re-feeding syndrome. Therefore, only a fraction of the patient's nutritional requirements, for example less than 50%, should be given initially. The PN regimen can then be gradually increased every two to three days until full nutritional support is achieved.

Prior to commencing PN, it is essential to gain as much information as possible to make an informed decision as to whether this is the most appropriate method of providing nutrition to a patient.

Patient assessment should include:

- a medical history
- allergy information
- the medical plan:
  o Why is PN required in preference to other means of provision (e.g. gastric or jejunal feeding)?
  o What is the expected duration of treatment (this may affect the type of central catheter required)?
  o What is the likely endpoint of treatment (is the patient expected to eat normally once they have recovered from bowel surgery or is their illness terminal, in which case consideration needs to be given as to whether the provision of PN is the most appropriate method of providing nutrition at this stage of their life)?
- Does the patient have suitable dedicated access? If no access is available:
  o Are there arrangements in hand for a central catheter to be inserted?
  o What type of central catheter is planned?
  o Is a multi-lumen catheter required for multiple treatments?
  o When will the procedure take place?
- weight since admission (or recent weight) where possible
- recent bloods
- when the person last received adequate nutrition

- fluid-balance issues; appropriately completed fluid-balance charts (for the previous 24–48 hrs) can be of some use
- Does the patient require additional intravenous fluid infusions? This may have an affect on the volume of PN that can be prescribed.

Once these issues have been discussed and the course of treatment agreed, it is considered good practice, where possible, to tell the patient why IV feeding is required, and what its potential risks and benefits are.

Weight

Weight is an integral requirement for most nutrient-requirement calculations. It allows an estimate of a patient's nutritional requirements, even in its simplest form of 25–35 kcal/kg of body weight, and is also used as a guide for fluid requirements. In planned admissions for surgical procedures, you should expect to find a weight from pre-assessment clinic, or out-patient clinic, as weights are required for anaesthetic purposes. Often, patients will have an idea of what their usual weight is, or what their most recent weight was. This can then be used as a baseline. It is important to remember that weight can be affected by oedema and ascites.

Height

The patient's height should be recorded to enable the calculation of their body mass index (BMI). Again, this may be recorded in medical notes from previous out-patient appointments. Many people do know what their height is, although they have a tendency to be optimistic!

Bloods

Recent bloods are essential to establish a baseline prior to commencing nutrition support. They should include liver-function tests (LFTs), urea and electrolytes (U & Es), magnesium, phosphate, calcium and full blood count (FBC).

In order to establish whether the patient is at risk of re-feeding syndrome, it is useful to identify how long the patient has been without adequate nutrition. If it has been some time (more than seven days), then the patient will be at risk of developing re-feeding syndrome once PN is commenced. This may influence the amount of nutrition support provided. NICE (2006) advises that PN should be introduced 'progressively' and monitored closely, usually giving no more than 50% estimated requirements for the first 24–48 hours. In practice, it is sensible to commence PN feeding with the smallest available ready-made bag, providing approximately 1000 kcal, and 5 g nitrogen. If it was felt that this was too much nutrition for a patient to cope with, a part of this bag could be given. Pabrinex (intravenous B and C vitamins) is usually administered prior to administration of PN for the first three days, to help reduce the risk of re-feeding syndrome (see Chapter 7 for further details on re-feeding syndrome).

Routes for intravenous access

The provision of PN requires intravenous access through a dedicated line. The type of access used will depend on a number of factors, including the length of time PN is required, the availability of suitable veins, the level of expertise of the staff inserting the line and patient choice.

If PN is only required for a relatively short period of time, i.e. up to seven days, an existing central venous catheter (CVC) may be used to save the patient having to undergo another procedure. In such cases, it is not always necessary to flush the line with antibiotics prior to starting PN. However, check your policies/infection-control department for local information.

A number of veins are suitable to provide central access for PN.

Subclavian vein

The subclavian route is often the preferred route for long-term PN, i.e. lasting over 30 days (National Institute for Health and Clinical Excellence, 2006). However, as there is an associated risk of pneumothorax during the insertion procedure, the jugular route is often used in preference for short-term administration. There is a lower risk of infection associated with using the subclavian route as the exit point for a subclavian catheter lies between the sternum and the nipple, allowing the catheter to be safely secured to the chest wall, thereby reducing movement, increasing patient comfort and reducing the number of dressing changes required.

Jugular vein

Whilst the insertion of a CVC through the jugular vein is associated with a lower risk of complication, there is an increased risk of infection post insertion owing to the position of the exit site on the neck.

Dressing application is often more difficult, and more frequent dressing replacements are required because of movement of the neck during normal daily activities and hair growth (particularly a problem for men). The position of the catheter may also make head movement uncomfortable for the patient as a pulling sensation is felt. For these reasons, jugular access is not recommended for the administration of PN beyond five to seven days (Hamilton, 2000).

Basilic and cephalic veins

Accessing the basilic or cephalic veins carries a much lower complication rate during insertion of a CVC and a lower infection risk post insertion. Dressing application is easy and routine changes are usually required only on a weekly basis. However, in the acutely ill patient these veins prove difficult to gain access to, especially to the inexperienced operator, owing to previous cannulations, repeated blood tests or oedema.

Femoral vein

Wherever possible, the femoral route should be avoided for PN. Owing to the position of the exit point of the catheter, the use of the femoral vein carries a high risk of infection and thrombosis. There is also a much higher demand for nursing management of skin hygiene because of the risk of contamination at the catheter site from urine and faeces. Dressing application may also be an issue, particularly in patients who are mobile or incontinent, as frequent dressing changes will be required.

Types of central venous catheter

The type of catheter used will depend upon the length of time PN is required and the condition of the patient's veins. Many infusion mixtures are hypertonic and can therefore only be administered through veins with a high blood flow, i.e. the central veins.

A planned approach to central venous access is required in patients who are likely to require longer periods of PN to minimise the need for repeated insertions of shorter-term catheters.

Non-tunnelled central venous catheters

A short-term catheter is one that is inserted directly into the central circulation, usually via the jugular or subclavian vein. They may also be inserted into the femoral vein, but as already identified this route is not recommended for the administration of PN.

They are usually made from polyurethane, making it less pliable than silicone devices, which increases the risk of irritation of the inner lumen of the vessel accessed and is more thrombogenic (Springhouse Corporation, 2002).

This type of device can be single- or multi-lumen, giving the option to administer multiple therapies through one device. It is suitable for use for up to 14 days (Dougherty & Lister, 2008).

Peripherally inserted central catheter

A peripherally inserted central catheter (PICC) is made of silicone and inserted into the basilic or cephalic vein in the antecubital fossa. It is advanced into the central circulation so the tip sits within the lower third of the superior vena cava (Todd, 1998; Royal College of Nursing, 2005) and is therefore suitable for the administration of hyperosmolar feeds. It should not be confused with a midclavicular catheter, or 'long line', where the tip of the catheter sits in one of the veins leading to the superior vena cava, such as the subclavian or proximal axillary vein (Carlson, 1999).

To ensure the successful placement of a PICC, careful assessment of the patient's veins should take place before insertion is attempted. The patient should have good-size veins that can be clearly identified and that have not been exposed to repeated cannulation attempts. The basilic and cephalic veins may be smaller in female patients and so consideration will need to be given to the size of the central catheter inserted to minimise the risk of phlebitis developing following insertion.

There are a number of advantages to using a PICC:

- It can be placed at the patient's bedside, increasingly by nursing staff who have been appropriately trained.
- It has a lower complication rate associated with the insertion procedure than central lines.
- It is associated with a lower infection rate once inserted.

Therefore, its placement should be considered as a first option and not only when all attempts at providing more traditional central catheter placements have failed. If cared for properly, a PICC can be used for the administration of PN for a number of months, proving to be a suitable alternative for other types of central access.

However, the insertion of a PICC may be more difficult or contra-indicated in patients who present with:

- marked hypercatabolism that need increased energy and protein requirements
- severe burns
- inadequate antecubital fossa veins
- veins that are compromised by oedema
- a pre-existing skin infection
- uncorrected coagulopathy
- anatomical distortions.
(Timmis, 1998; Todd, 1998; Palmer & McFie, 2001)

Tunnelled central venous catheters

A tunnelled CVC is the most appropriate access for patients requiring long-term PN as it is associated with a lower rate of catheter colonisation (National Institute for Health and Clinical Excellence, 2006).

The subclavian vein is usually used. The line lies in a subcutaneous tunnel before entering a central vein and usually exits at some point between the sternum and the nipple. The device is made of silicone with a Dacron cuff attached. The Dacron cuff allows the development of fibrosis within the tunnelled segment, minimising the need to provide a means of external fixation, thus reducing patient discomfort and the need for repeated dressing changes.

The insertion of a tunnelled CVC is a surgical procedure and insertion should be carried out in a theatre, radiology or ultrasound department.

Implantable access device

Although not commonly used, another alternative in the provision of long-term central access is the use of an implantable device. It can be used as an alternative to central line placement for those patients who require frequent intravenous access for at least three months (Schummer *et al.*, 2003). It may be an option for those patients who require PN but are running out of accessible veins or are conscious about their body image. An implanted port consists of a reservoir with a self-sealing septum which is attached to a silicone catheter. It is usually inserted into the subclavian or cephalic vein.

Non-central access options

Peripheral cannula

As its name suggests, a peripheral cannula sits in a peripheral vein. A small peripheral cannula (normally used for the administration of IV fluids) is normally only used to administer PN when other means of providing central or peripheral access have been exhausted or are deemed unsuitable.

Although easy to insert, the use of a peripheral cannula for PN will limit the type of solution administered, require repeated interventions from healthcare staff and is associated with a risk of thrombophlebitis. The development of thrombophlebitis is caused by the administration of hypertonic parenteral solutions through small veins, causing irritation (Bandregt & Soeters, 2005). To minimise this risk, the cannula should be placed in one of the larger veins in the forearm and re-sited every 48 hours according to patient need and availability of veins. If a peripheral cannula is to be used, NICE (2006) recommends the use of a 22–23 fr (ch) cannula. This type of access should only be used for short-term administration of PN as it often causes distress to the patient, is time-consuming for healthcare professionals and will only tolerate the administration of a fraction of the patient's total nutritional requirements.

Midline

This type of vascular access is not usually recommended for the administration of PN, because, similar to a peripheral cannula, mechanical phlebitis can be a problem. It may be used as an option in patients where insertion of a central line is contraindicated and where peripheral access is difficult.

A midline catheter is made of either polyurethane or silicone, varies in length from 7.5 cm to 20 cm (Carlson, 1999; Perucca, 2001) and is inserted into the antecubital fossa, but, unlike a PICC, see above, its tip sits in the veins of the upper arm and does not enter the central circulation.

As the tip of a peripheral cannula or midline catheter does not sit in the central circulation, there is a restriction on the type of feeding solution that can be administered through them, as not all regimens are suitable for peripheral administration. Hypocaloric or low-osmolality feed can be administered, but it is important to note that the patient's full nutritional requirements may not be met via this route.

Multi-lumen vs single-lumen catheters

Multi-lumen central catheters can be used for a combination of treatments such as chemotherapy, antibiotic therapy and PN. Some reports highlight the risk of an increased incidence of catheter-related sepsis with multi-lumen lines (Pemberton *et al.*, 1986; McCarthy *et al.*, 1987). The counterargument is that there is no statistical difference in catheter-related sepsis between using single- or triple-lumen catheters (Johnson & Rypins, 1990; Farkas *et al.*, 1992; Goetz *et al.*, 1998).

It is, however, considered best practice that if central access is only required for the administration of PN a single-lumen catheter should be used. If the patient is acutely ill and a multi-lumen line is essential for the provision of a number of treatments, one lumen must be reserved for the administration of PN only and should be clearly labelled to prevent the administration of other therapies or the withdrawal of blood.

Confirming central venous catheter tip position

Once a CVC has been successfully inserted, the distal tip should sit in the lower third of the superior vena cava or right atrium (Royal College of Nursing, 2005; Hamilton, 2006; National Institute for Health and Clinical Excellence, 2006). Tip placement should be confirmed with a chest X-ray or ultrasonic locating device (National Institute for Health and Clinical Excellence, 2006) prior to the administration of PN.

Using a previously used central venous catheter

In some instances, referral for PN will be received in patients who already have a central line for other treatments. In such cases, as long as there is a free lumen which can be dedicated to the administration of PN, it may be in the best interests of the patient to use it, particularly if this avoids the need for further line insertions in the short term. If all lumens have been used for other treatments, it is acceptable to use a previously used lumen, providing it has been flushed with saline. The use of flushing or locking a central line lumen with antibiotics prior to the administration of PN is no longer considered necessary.

Aftercare of line and insertion site

Non-tunnelled central venous catheters

These catheters are held in place with external sutures. A transparent dressing is usually placed over the insertion site to minimise infection risks. The site should be observed daily but the dressing should be disturbed as little as possible unless a dressing change is clinically indicated, for example when the dressing becomes loose or there is exudate around the exit site.

If left in for extended periods, the catheter material may cause irritation on the inner lumen of the vessel.

Peripherally inserted central catheter

Peripherally inserted central catheters (PICCs) are designed with suture wings which can be used to suture the PICC to the patient's skin. Some have the suture wings attached directly to the tube; others may need to be fitted following placement. One disadvantage of using sutures is that long-term suturing can be uncomfortable for the patient (Gabriel, 2000, 2001). They may also cause scarring once the device is removed.

A PICC can be adequately secured using sterile adhesive strips positioned close to the exit point of the catheter plus a self-adhesive security device. These have been shown to significantly increase the length of time a PICC remains in position and reduces the incidence of complications (Sheppard *et al.*, 1999). Once secured, the insertion site is covered with a moisture-permeable transparent dressing, which should be changed only as clinically indicated.

When using these measures in preference to suturing, the careful removal of the transparent dressing is required to prevent dislodging the PICC during dressing changes. It is not unknown for a PICC to become dislodged from the central vein through an overly vigorous dressing removal.

Tunnelled lines

It normally takes between six and seven days for the skin tunnel to heal following insertion. Once healed, the entry site sutures can be removed. Fibrosis around the Dacron cuff may take up to a further two weeks to develop, during which time the sutures at the exit site should not be removed. The development of a fibrin sheath around the Dacron cuff is essential to ensure the long-term security of the

CVC (Stacey *et al.*, 1991; Weinstein, 2001; Perucca, 2001). A transparent dressing should be placed over the site and changed weekly or as clinically indicated until the exit site sutures are removed. Once the exit site sutures have been removed, there is no further need for the application of a dressing, unless requested by the patient.

Implantable port

As this device is implanted subcutaneously, care of the site is minimal when not in use. When used, the needle can remain in situ for up to a week (Springhouse Corporation, 2002). Frequent needle insertions to gain access to the device can cause discomfort, especially in the early stages of use. Where this occurs, a local anaesthetic cream can be useful. Over time, the tissue affected can become scarred and the patient may experience a loss of sensitivity (Perucca, 2001).

As with any other central access device, there should be a regular assessment of the site to monitor for signs of infection, extravasation or needle dislodgement.

Peripheral cannula

The peripheral cannula is normally secured with a transparent dressing which should not need replacing as the line will only be in situ for two days.

Regular observations of the site should be undertaken to detect early signs of thrombophlebitis. The application of a heat pad placed directly above the cannula can prove useful in minimising the development of thrombophlebitis. Application is usually required three or four times a day for at least 15–20 minutes over the first 24–48 hours. Alternatively, the use of a glyceryl trinitrate (GTN) patch applied distal to the cannula may also prove useful.

Midline

These devices can be secured using sterile adhesive strips plus a self-adhesive security device. The exit site should then be covered with a sterile transparent dressing and changed as clinically indicated.

Dressing changes

When changing a dressing on any CVC, a strict aseptic technique must be maintained. Sterile gloves must be worn and a sterile dressing pack used. The insertion site must be inspected each time the line is accessed for signs of erythema, tenderness, swelling or exudate.

A chlorhexidine solution should be used to clean the site. Maki *et al.* (1991) found chlorhexidine 2% aqueous solution to be the most effective. The use of chlorhexidine in preference to povidone iodine was also supported by Garland *et al.* (1995), Danks (2006) and Mimoz *et al.* (2007).

For short-term CVCs, PICCs and newly inserted tunnelled catheters a water-permeable transparent film dressing should be used to cover the exit site, ensuring that the site is completely covered and evenly applied. A transparent dressing may be left in situ for up to seven days but should be changed more frequently if it becomes wet, soiled or no longer intact (Dougherty & Lister, 2008). This is to minimise the possibility of introducing bacterial contamination. The use of sterile gauze dressings should not be encouraged unless clinically indicated for a number of reasons (Box 6.1).

Box 6.1   Advantages and disadvantages of dressing options for CVCs

Transparent dressings	Gauze dressings
• The dressing used must be moisture-permeable. • Using a non-moisture-permeable dressing will increase the level of moisture at the exit site and hence increase the risk of infection. • Once in place, these dressings can be left in situ for up to seven days. (Therefore, they reduce the number of manipulations required at the site and reduce the risk of bacterial contamination.) • A bandage should not be used to cover a transparent dressing, as it reduces visibility and the moisture-permeability of the dressing.	• Inability to visualise the site without disturbing the dressing. • More frequent dressing changes are required, at least daily. May be more frequent if the dressing becomes soiled as it is unable to provide a barrier against bacteria and water, thus increasing the risk of contamination. • Increased manipulations at the exit site increase the risk of infection. • Tape securing the gauze dressing can become loose, leaving the exit site exposed.

Therefore, the ideal dressing would be

- transparent:
  - to allow visual inspection of the catheter and catheter site
- self-adhesive:
  - to provide greater stability
  - to reduce the risk of trauma and mechanical phlebitis
  - to reduce the risk of bacterial contamination
- semi-permeable:
  - to allow the site to 'breathe'
- sterile.

Observations

Owing to the risks associated with CVC insertion, the patient must be monitored to detect signs of complications, particularly in the first 24 hours following insertion (Table 6.1). Therefore, the frequent moni-

Table 6.1　Potential complications following insertion of a CVC

Time	Observe for
Immediate post op period	• pyrexia • tachycardia • hypotension • vomiting • shoulder pain • changes in respiratory function • feeling generally unwell especially if this problem coincides with the placement of the catheter or following initial administration of PN. Vital signs should be monitored at least hourly for the first six hours.
Up to three days' post insertion	• pneumothorax (when the subclavian vein is accessed) • catheter misplacement. Vital signs should be monitored every four to six hours.
Ongoing monitoring	• pyrexia • tachycardia • hypotension • inflammation, exudate or discomfort around exit site of catheter. Vital signs should be monitored every four to six hours.

toring of vital signs and observation of the development of symptoms are essential.

Flushing following insertion

Immediately following insertion, a CVC is normally flushed with a heparin solution to minimise the risk of platelet aggregation.

On a daily basis, the frequency of flushing and the type of solution used will depend upon the type of catheter in use, for example a valved PICC is usually flushed once a week with a 0.9% sodium chloride solution, whilst an open-ended PICC should be flushed with a heparinised solution (Dougherty & Lister, 2008). If in doubt, consult the manufacturer's recommendations and your local guidelines.

Peripheral cannula, midline and non-tunnelled central lines should be flushed following each use with 0.9% sodium chloride solution.

Estimating nutritional requirements

Nutritional requirements for adults requiring nutrition support are usually estimated by dietitians using the Schofield equations. These are based on age and weight, and are used to estimate their basal metabolic rate (BMR). Stress factors, for example bowel surgery, are then added in, if appropriate, as is an adjustment for weight loss or gain. An activity factor is then added, which combines with the energy required to metabolise the feed (diet-induced thermogenesis, or DIT).

When estimating nutritional requirements, it is recommended that the lower end of the range is used initially. This should be monitored regularly, and amended if necessary (Soulsby & Weekes, 2004). Owing to the risks of overfeeding, and re-feeding syndrome, it is always safer to start with smaller amounts of nutrition and increase gradually. Much is still unknown about the optimum amount of nutrition required in illness.

When prescribing PN, together with energy and nitrogen, decisions need to be made regarding other electrolytes – sodium, potassium, calcium, magnesium and phosphate – and total fluid volume.

For those who are not severely ill or injured, or at risk of re-feeding syndrome, normal PN prescriptions would usually provide:

- 25–35 kcal/kg/day total energy
- 0.13–0.24 g/nitrogen/kg/day
- 30–35 ml fluid/kg
- sufficient electrolytes, minerals and micronutrients (National Institute for Health and Clinical Excellence, 2006).

In seriously ill, injured or in individuals at risk of re-feeding syndrome, PN should be administered cautiously, generally starting at no more than half the estimated energy and protein needs, building up as clinical condition allows.

Biochemical and haematological assessment

Biochemical and haematological tests are required to establish baseline levels prior to starting PN, and then to monitor the effect of the therapy.

The following tests are required before starting PN:

- sodium
- potassium
- calcium
- magnesium
- phosphate
- urea
- creatinine
- bilirubin
- alkaline phosphatase
- alanine aminotransferase (ALT)
- total protein
- albumin.

In specific cases, it may also be appropriate to measure levels of trace elements, for example zinc, but the results may not be available for a week or more if these tests are not carried out on site.

During the first week of PN, these blood tests should be repeated daily. During the second week of PN the frequency of monitoring may be reduced to three times a week if the patient's condition is stable. During subsequent weeks of PN, twice-weekly monitoring may be sufficient.

Preparations available

Two different types of PN preparations are available: standard ready-made bags and tailored PN bags, which are usually formulated in a pharmacy's aseptic unit.

Standard bags

A standard bag of PN has the advantage of being easy to prepare. Each manufacturer provides a range of bags containing fixed amounts of protein, lipids and calories. Each bag also contains a baseline level of electrolytes which can be topped up to meet individual patient requirements in the pharmacy's aseptic unit, if necessary. Standard bags are not suitable for every patient; so each patient should be assessed by a Nutrition Support Team as special prescriptions may be required.

Tailored bags

A tailored bag is made up from scratch usually by specialised pharmacists. The ingredients (protein, carbohydrate, fat, electrolytes and vitamins) are all compounded separately following compatibility checks. This is usually a far lengthier process than that performed for standard bags, but is useful if an ingredient needs to be omitted (for example when producing lipid-free PN).

Nutritional content of parenteral nutrition

Protein

The protein content of PN is normally expressed as grams of nitrogen. Nitrogen is normally supplied as a mixture of essential and non-essential amino acids. The optimum amino acid profile for PN is still unknown (Thomas & Bishop, 2007).

Energy

Energy is provided in the form of glucose together with lipid (see below). Different concentrations of glucose can be used depending on the total volume of PN required. If high concentrations of glucose are compounded (i.e. over 10% glucose), the solution is more concentrated. It cannot therefore be administered peripherally. Where this type of PN is required a central line must be used.

Fat

Fat emulsions are commonly long-chain triglycerides (LCTs) and essential fatty acids. Medium-chain triglycerides (MCTs) are rapidly metabolised and can be combined with LCTs in PN. This has the advantage of faster clearance from the plasma and reduces accumulation (Murphy & Scott, 2000). Some newer PN products contain olive oil or fish-oil based lipids. Fat normally provides between 30% and 50% of the calories contained in PN and helps reduce the risk of hyperglycaemia common with glucose-only regimens (Thomas & Bishop, 2007).

Fluid

Fluid is an essential part of PN therapy and needs to be carefully adjusted according to the patient's fluid balance. Bags usually contain between one and three litres of fluid. It is possible to add extra fluid to PN if required for patients with exceptional fluid losses, although for most patients if additional fluid is required concurrent administration of IV fluids is used.

Electrolytes

Electrolytes can be added to PN preparations to provide adequate maintenance or to correct deficiencies, for example:

- magnesium
- phosphate
- sodium
- potassium
- calcium.

Vitamins and trace elements

Vitamins and trace elements are not routinely included in standard bags and should, therefore, always be added. Any additions made should be carried out in controlled pharmaceutical conditions – not at ward level (National Institute for Health and Clinical Excellence, 2006). Trace-element additives tend to be either Additrace (Fresenius Kabi) or Decan (Baxter).

Water-soluble vitamins are contained in Solivito N (Fresenius Kabi), with fat-soluble vitamins contained in Vitlipid N (Fresenius Kabi). Cernevit (Baxter) contains a combination of fat- and water-soluble vitamins, but does not contain vitamin K, which needs to be administered separately, if appropriate.

Vitamins and trace elements are usually added to the PN as close to administration as possible, to prevent interactions and to minimise any possibility of absorption of fat-soluble vitamins onto the plastic bag and infusion set.

Glutamine

Glutamine is recognised as a conditionally essential amino acid in catabolic states. Glutamine levels are known to drop after major surgery and during critical illness. Lower levels are associated with immune dysfunction and higher mortality. Evidence for its use is still inconclusive and the optimum dose is still unknown (Sains, 2005). Glutamine can be incorporated into PN for patients satisfying specific criteria on local protocols. It may be considered for patients who are malnourished and have undergone major gastrointestinal surgery.

Allergies to components of parenteral nutrition

Some ranges of PN use egg phospholipids and soybean oils to which patients may have allergic reactions. Known hypersensitivity to egg or soy protein or to any of the excipients will mean the administration of PN is contraindicated and an alternative product will need to be prescribed.

Drug therapy that may affect nutrition support

The patient's medication history and current drug prescription should be reviewed before starting PN and at intervals while the patient continues on PN. The patient's drug therapy may provide clues as to the patient's nutritional status, may indicate that additional monitoring is required or may affect the nutrition support provided.

For example:

- diuretics: close monitoring of U & E results and fluid balance
- antidiabetic agents or insulin: close monitoring of blood-sugar levels and potassium; may predispose to re-feeding syndrome

- cardiovascular or respiratory disease: close monitoring of fluid balance
- vitamin, mineral or electrolyte supplements: close monitoring of levels and doses
- gastrointestinal agents: consider possible malabsorption
- metronidazole infusion 500 mg 8-hourly: provides 300 ml fluid and 45 mmol sodium per day
- propofol infusion: provides 1 kcal/ml
- drug infusions in 0.9% sodium chloride: contains 15 mmol sodium per 100 ml
- drug infusions in 5% glucose: contains 5 g glucose and 20 kcal per 100 ml
- total volume of IV drugs and flushes compared with the patient's fluid requirement: multiple antibiotic infusions soon add up to a significant volume.

Care of parenteral nutrition before administration

When PN is delivered to the clinical area, it should be stored at a temperature of 4–8 °C. A designated refrigerator for storage of PN or the ward drug refrigerator is ideal for storage. Appropriate storage is particularly important if more than one bag is delivered to the clinical area (for example to ensure adequate supply over a weekend or bank holidays or for multiple patients).

Where PN is stored in a refrigerator, it should be removed approximately one hour before its intended use to allow the feed to settle and warm through to room temperature (Royal College of Nursing, 2005). The bag should not be artificially warmed by placing directly in warm water or placing over direct heat (Hardy & Sizer, 1999). Do not handle the bag unnecessarily or shake it. Failure to allow the bag to settle before use will prevent bubbles within the solution dispersing. This may result in bubbles remaining within the feed, which as it is administered through the giving set will cause the pump to alarm; this is particularly annoying during overnight feeding.

No additions should be made to a bag of PN by staff at ward level. Each bag will have been tailored to meet the individual patient's requirements with specific electrolytes added dependent on the patient's biochemistry results.

If there appears to be any leakage from the bag of feed or giving set or either appears to have been tampered with, do not use the affected bag. Inform the prescribing team and the pharmacy department.

A coloured plastic bag usually accompanies the first batch of PN delivered to the clinical area from pharmacy. It should be placed over the bag to be administered as it is being hung on the IV stand at the patient's bedside. The coloured bag is required to protect the vitamin A content of the infusion. Vitamin A is light-sensitive and degradation may occur if the bag of PN is exposed to ultraviolet light found in sunlight (Hardy & Sizer, 1999). Therefore, it is important to ensure that if PN is administered during the day it is not positioned close to windows. Exposure to artificial light does not cause the same level of degradation, but nevertheless the cover is a useful safety precaution.

For the patient receiving PN the IV administration sets should be changed every 24 hours (Department of Health, 2001; Gillies *et al.*, 2004; Royal College of Nursing, 2005) and immediately if contamination is suspected or where the integrity of the system has been compromised (Royal College of Nursing, 2005). Some hospitals will arrange to have the giving sets attached to the bag of PN in pharmacy whilst they are making vitamin and electrolyte additions in a sterile environment. If this is not the case and it is necessary to attach the giving set to the bag of PN in the clinical area, a protocol should be agreed within the organisation and a strict aseptic technique must apply during the procedure. Once the giving set is attached to the bag of PN and it is taken out of the refrigerator, the feed should not be used for longer than 24 hours (Burnham, 1999; Wilson, 2001), although some areas start the patient's nutrition regimen with a bag of PN administered over 48 hours. If a bag of PN is discontinued for therapy or surgery extending beyond one hour, the bag should not be re-used; it should be discarded.

A volumetric pump must be used to ensure accurate administration of the PN according to the rate prescribed.

The rate of feed should not be adjusted without consultation with the prescriber/Nutrition Support Team, as the regimen agreed will have been calculated to meet the patient's nutritional requirements for a specified period, usually 24 hours. Some acutely ill patients may be medically unable to cope with a more rapid infusion of feed especially if it is unregulated. Before rates of feed are adjusted, other factors in the patient's treatment will need to be considered, such as whether the patient is receiving additional IV fluids or electrolytes. It thus becomes clear why unlike a bag of enteral feed PN should only be used for the patient for whom it is prescribed and at the rate prescribed.

Mode of delivery: continuous or cyclical administration

PN is usually administered in the early stages by continuous infusion over 24 hours. NICE (2006) states that continuous administration of PN should be the preferred method of infusion in severely ill patients who require PN. The change towards cyclical administration should be gradual, but should be considered in patients requiring PN for more than two weeks.

Some patients, however, may benefit from different infusion periods in order to facilitate their recovery. For instance, PN infused over 18 hours with a six-hour break during the day frees the patient from attachments, which may facilitate more effective physiotherapy sessions. The change from continuous to cyclical administration should only be made once the patient's regimen is stable, and with the agreement of the patient (as the additional fluid input during the night affects urine output and often disrupts the patient's sleep). If cyclical administration is used, nursing staff must take extra precautions to flush the central line as soon as the PN infusion finishes, and again before it is re-commenced, to reduce the risk of line blockage.

Administration of medication through a central venous catheter

No medication should be given through a lumen on a central line required for PN or through the ports on the giving set. PN is incompatible with a number of medications (Dougherty & Lister, 2008) and may increase the risk of catheter occlusion. No medication should be administered into the bag of PN once it is being infused (Royal College of Nursing, 2005). If additional medications, fluids or electrolytes are required, they should be administered through a separate lumen or a peripheral cannula.

Should an in-line filter be used?

The aim of an in-line filter is to prevent the administration of enlarged lipid droplets, fungal contaminants and inadvertent particulate debris from entering the giving set and hence the CVC. The filter is attached to the base of the bag of PN and the tip of the giving set.

Fungal contamination should not be an issue as the preparation of PN is under aseptic conditions within a sterile compounding unit and therefore is not an indication for the use of filters. Hamilton (2000) highlights the risk of thrombophlebitis resulting from particles and additives in the feed, which the use of a filter has been shown to reduce. However, opinion on the benefit of using a filter is divided. NICE (2003) states that in-line filters should not be used routinely for infection prevention purposes in PN, whilst *Standards for Infusion Therapy* (Royal College of Nursing, 2005) recommends that in-line filtration should be used.

The use of a filter is not without additional cost. In patients receiving short-term PN through a multi-lumen CVC with additional IV infusions without in-line filters, the additional cost may not be justified.

Maintaining catheter patency

Flushing is essential to minimise the risk of occlusion even where the administration of PN is continuous. The CVC must be flushed before starting the infusion and on completion of a bag. Sterile normal saline is usually used. It is advisable to use a rapid push/pause technique to administer the saline as it creates turbulence within the lumen dislodging any build-up of particles that may occur, decreasing the risk of occlusion before locking the line. If a feed is stopped for any reason, the lumen must be flushed immediately. Use a 10 ml syringe or larger. Smaller syringes will increase the pressure exerted upon the catheter, potentially leading to venous damage or rupture of the lumen. An aseptic technique must be used.

Patient monitoring

As many patients receiving PN are often critically ill or immunocompromised, regular and timely monitoring of the patient is essential to ensure the nutritional support provided meets the patient's requirements and to detect signs of complications at the earliest possible stage. In the initial stages, monitoring should be frequent. Fluid balance, biochemical markers, blood glucose and anthropometric measurements should be measured regularly. Once the patient is established on a regimen and is biochemically stable, the frequency of monitoring can be reduced.

Fluid balance

Strict records of fluid intake and output are vital to ensure accurate calculations are made of the patient's fluid requirements and to avoid fluid overload or dehydration. It is essential to record not only urinary output but to include fluid loss through vomiting, diarrhoea, gastric aspirate and fistula output. Fluid-balance charts should be interpreted in conjunction with the patient's weight where possible.

Fluid-balance charts when completed accurately also serve to compare the volume of feed prescribed with the actual volume of feed delivered or received. Clear documentation of other documented IV/ enteral fluid infusions will allow the Nutrition Support Team to calculate the energy and/or electrolyte content of these fluids, which will be taken into consideration when calculating the level of PN required.

Additional intravenous fluids may be required in patients who have a high-output fistula, but if total fluid intake is not clearly recorded this may result in fluid overload if the fluid content provided by PN is not taken into consideration. To minimise this risk, ensure the patient's medical team is aware of the fluid provided through PN and clearly record all fluid intake and output on fluid charts and in the relevant patient notes.

Biochemistry

As with enteral feeding, regular biochemical monitoring is essential. However, unlike enteral feeding which uses pre-prepared feeds, there is much more flexibility in making additions to a bag of PN, tailoring it to meet an individual's requirements.

Urea and electrolytes

Monitor daily until stable, then twice weekly.
  Check:

- sodium, to assess hydration status use in conjunction with the fluid-balance chart to interpret results; observe for signs of over- or under-hydration
- potassium, to detect abnormalities (metabolic or electrolyte) and for monitoring of re-feeding syndrome
- urea, to assess hydration status
- creatinine, to monitor renal function.

Liver-function tests

Establish baseline then monitor twice weekly until stable, then weekly.

LFTs can detect:

- hepatic dysfunction, which is common in PN-fed patients
- overfeeding.

Albumin

Low-serum albumin levels are associated with a high risk of morbidity and mortality, and may therefore help identify those in need of nutrition support, but are of limited value in monitoring PN, owing to long half life, and its extracellular distribution. This makes it more indicative of hydration status and clinical condition than nutritional status.

Phosphate, magnesium and calcium

Establish baseline, then monitor daily if at risk of re-feeding syndrome, three times a week until stable and then weekly.

- **Phosphate and magnesium:** depletion is common and often goes undetected; regular monitoring is essential to detect re-feeding syndrome.
- **Calcium:** needs to be corrected for serum albumin concentration. Hypo- or hypercalcaemia may occur. Hypocalcaemia may be secondary to magnesium deficiency.

C-Reactive protein

Establish baseline then monitor twice-weekly. This is to assess for the presence of an acute phase reaction. A one-off result is of little use. It is the trend of results that is important. CRP assists in the interpretation of protein, trace element and vitamin results.

White cell count

Establish baseline then monitor twice-weekly to detect infection or sepsis.

Haemoglobin and mean corpuscular volume

Establish baseline then monitor twice-weekly until stable, then weekly to detect anaemia. A deficiency of iron or folate is fairly common.

In practice, whilst other monitoring is desirable (such as selenium, zinc and copper) we have found it difficult to get timely results, often with patients completing their course of PN before their results are confirmed. However, in long-term PN, these would need to be monitored on a regular basis. Zinc and copper should be monitored every two to four weeks. Deficiency is common, particularly if a patient has wounds and/or high gastrointestinal losses.

NICE (2006) guidelines have further information regarding additional biochemical monitoring for long-term PN.

Blood glucose

Blood glucose should be monitored at least daily to indicate whether changes in the PN feeding regimen or blood-glucose control (for example insulin) are necessary.

Hyperglycaemia may occur because of carbohydrate overload or stress-induced insulin resistance (Dougherty & Lister, 2008). Until stabilised, the use of a sliding-scale insulin regimen may be necessary. Failure to recognise the symptoms of hyperglycaemia can result in osmotic diuresis, which may contribute to urinary-tract infections and weight loss. Maintenance of normoglycaemia with insulin reduces mortality and morbidity of critically ill patients (Van den Berghe *et al.*, 2003).

Complications associated with the administration of parenteral nutrition

There are a number of complications that may occur with the administration of PN which may be of a mechanical, metabolic or infectious nature. Some of the more common problems that may occur are discussed below.

Catheter-related problems

The administration of PN through a CVC provides an ideal environment for microbial growth. A high standard of catheter care is one of the most important factors in minimising the incidence of catheter-related infections.

Thrombophlebitis

This complication is usually associated with peripheral access. It can be painful, making the vein unusable for a period. The patient may show signs of erythema and inflammation and find it painful to move the affected arm. To minimise the risk of thrombophlebitis, the smallest possible cannula should be inserted into the largest available vein. This is why the use of PN through a peripheral vein is discouraged. To prevent thrombophlebitis, the use of a heat pad may prove effective (see the **Peripheral cannula** section above).

Exit-site infection

Exit-site infection is usually recognised by inflammation, exudate and pain directly around the exit site of a central line.

A wound swab should be taken, antibiotics commenced and the site cleaned thoroughly using an aseptic technique as per hospital policy. Check that the site is covered with the appropriate sterile dressing and disturbance of the site is reduced to a minimum.

Tunnel infection

This type of infection can be identified by signs of inflammation along the line of the catheter beyond the exit site. It cannot be as easily treated as an exit-site infection and may result in removal of the line. A swab should be taken of the exit site and bloods taken directly from the CVC and from peripheral veins for culture.

If a short-term CVC is in use, consider removing the line. A period of 24 hours must lapse, during which time appropriate IV antibiotics are administered before the insertion of another central line.

If a long-term catheter is in place, take swabs at the exit site, peripheral and central line blood cultures and commence appropriate IV antibiotics.

Catheter-related sepsis

This is a far more serious type of infection. The patient presents with pyrexia and rigors particularly after the infusion commences. It is important to determine that the central line is the cause of the infection and that the patient does not have any other foci of sepsis. Central line and peripheral blood cultures should be taken. If the central line is identified as the source of infection, PN should be stopped and IV antibiotics commenced. Dependent upon the results of the blood cultures, the central catheter may be re-used, especially if a tunnelled line was needed for long-term access or where the insertion of a new line would be very difficult or unfeasible. Before use, the catheter would need to be locked with the appropriate antibiotics. Where a short-term central catheter is in situ, it should be removed and the catheter tip sent for culture.

Occlusion

Occlusion is usually recognised when there is resistance to the administration of feed or fluid into the catheter or to the withdrawal of blood from the catheter. These can be for a number of reasons (Box 6.2) and may arise suddenly, or a gradual resistance may be noted over a number of days. Before suspecting the worst, check that the catheter is not kinked or twisted externally by the patient lying against it or because a clamp is closed.

If there is a suspicion that the occlusion is due to an internal kinking or twisting of the catheter, an X-ray should be sought.

A sudden occlusion can usually be attributed to the administration of medication or the development of a fibrin sheath. Gradual occlusion is usually associated with the administration of lipids and is more likely to be the cause if the catheter occludes a couple of weeks after PN has been commenced.

Regular flushing (according to the manufacturer's instructions) and careful catheter maintenance will reduce the risk of an occlusion developing.

Unblocking a CVC is not without risk and should only be undertaken by practitioners who have received training and are competent.

Box 6.2   Causes of catheter occlusion

1. Mechanical obstruction
2. Thrombosis
3. Precipitation of drugs
4. The development of a fibrin sheath at the tip of the catheter
5. A build-up of lipid deposits from the administration of PN
6. Poor flushing technique or inadequate flushing
7. Slow-running infusion

Catheter damage

Catheter damage is more likely to develop if excess force is used when flushing the catheter or flattening of the lumen following repeated use of the clamp (not on all central lines). Some lines do have repair kits (PICC or Hickman lines), but repairs should only be undertaken by appropriately qualified healthcare professionals. If catheter damage is detected, immediate action must be taken to secure the catheter below the damaged area to prevent the development of an air embolism or infection, and the appropriate healthcare professional should be informed.

'Pyrexia of unknown origin'

If the patient presents with pyrexia for which the source cannot be traced, the central line will often be blamed as the source of infection. Where there is doubt and to avoid needless line removal, blood cultures should be obtained through the CVC and from a peripheral vein.

Non-catheter-related problems

Sleep disturbance

Overnight administration of PN may cause sleep disturbance not only because of the frequency of monitoring required when the patient is acutely ill but also because of potential problems associated with the administration of PN. The volumetric pump may alarm if the catheter occludes as the patient moves in their sleep (more of a problem with a PICC) or because of air in the line (which may occur if the bag has not been warmed to room temperature and allowed to settle before administration).

Another common problem is that the patient may feel the need to urinate more frequently owing to the continuous infusion of fluid.

It may help if the patient is made aware of these problems and is advised to sleep for short periods throughout the day.

Deficiency in micronutrient status

The term 'micronutrients' includes two main classes of nutrient substances, both of which are required in the diet in very small amounts: the essential inorganic micronutrients (trace elements) and the essential organic micronutrients (vitamins).

Deficiencies in micronutrient status may occur in patients who are receiving long-term PN or those who have malabsorption problems (Hardy & Sizer, 1999). This is less of an issue for patients who are fed for shorter periods. Detecting deficiencies and the monitoring of micronutrient status can be difficult and, as mentioned earlier, it may take several days to receive the results of laboratory tests. In addition, there is only a small body of knowledge about requirements, especially in disease (Shenkin, 1995).

Patients requiring nutrition support may have an increased requirement for micronutrients, as there may already be a whole body deficit as a result of malabsorption or increased losses, or inadequate replacement. There may be a need for a greater intake in those who are unwell compared with healthy individuals. Although the amounts of micronutrients available in PN may be adequate for most people, there may be individuals who require additional supplementation. This is not too difficult in those water-soluble nutrients where there is a large safety margin between effectiveness and toxicity. This is not the case with fat-soluble vitamins and some trace elements, where there is a much narrower margin of safety, and a degree of caution is required to prevent overdose.

It is likely that the only micronutrients that require regular assessment are zinc, copper, selenium, iron and folate (Shenkin, 1995). Other micronutrients should be assessed only when there is a clinical need.

Intravenous administration of micronutrients bypasses the selective absorption that would normally occur in the gut, which could increase the risk of an overdose of micronutrients given intravenously.

Metabolic problems

A number of metabolic problems may occur with the continued administration of PN, including:

- **Hypertriglyceridaemia:** This is an elevation of triglycerides in the bloodstream caused by the liver's inability to cope with the level of fat supplied within the PN.
- **Hyperglycaemia:** Raised blood-sugar levels which may be exacerbated by a chromium deficiency, which, as discussed above, is difficult to measure or treat.
- **Hepatic disorders:** For example, steatosis, cholestasis, and gallstones.

Discontinuing parenteral nutrition

Patients who have been nil by mouth for some time are unlikely to tolerate an adequate enteral diet straight away, and the transition from parenteral to enteral nutrition should therefore be a gradual process. Abrupt cessation of PN may also result in rebound hypoglycaemia.

If a patient is changing from PN to enteral tube feeding (via a nasogastric tube or a gastrostomy) a dietitian can prescribe a feeding regimen and liaise with the Nutrition Support Team regarding reducing or stopping PN. The enteral tube feed will normally be commenced at a low rate, for example 10–20 ml/hr, increasing gradually to around 100 ml/hr depending on how well the feed is tolerated by the patient.

If a patient is changing from PN to an oral diet the Nutrition Support Team will normally supervise the initial stages of this process, and then refer the patient to the ward dietitian when it is safe to stop PN.

The transition from PN to an oral diet may progress as seen in Table 6.2.

Occasionally, PN may be stopped before adequate enteral nutrition has been established, owing to other issues such as catheter-related

Table 6.2   The transition from PN to an oral diet

Oral intake	Impact on PN regimen
Start sips of water	Continue PN
Gradually increase oral intake of water	Continue PN and monitor fluid balance
Progress to clear fluids, e.g. tea/coffee without milk, juice/squash, clear soup, jelly, and juice-based nutritional supplements	Continue PN and monitor fluid balance
Progress to light diet, e.g. includes milky drinks, more substantial soup, and soft, well-cooked, easily digested foods	Consider reducing PN if tolerating more than one nutritional supplement drink per day
If tolerating light diet	Reduce PN and continue to increase oral intake
If meeting more than half their nutritional intake enterally	Stop PN

Box 6.3   Indications for removal of a CVC

- Incorrect positioning following X-ray
- Thrombus formation
- Occlusion which cannot be removed
- A leaking or damaged catheter which cannot be repaired.
- Infection

complications. If enteral nutrition has been started, the risks of catheter replacement are not justified. In these situations, the patient's nutritional intake should be carefully monitored.

Removal of a central venous catheter

CVCs should be removed as soon as possible after the discontinuation of PN, providing there is no further clinical need. There may be a number of other reasons why a CVC will need to be removed before the completion of treatment (Box 6.3), which will need to be assessed on an individual patient basis. Owing to the risk of complications associated with the removal of a CVC, PICCs and short-term CVCs can be removed at ward level according to local hospital policies and by registered nursing staff who are appropriately trained and competent (Royal College of Nursing, 2005); however, within most hospitals long-term tunnelled central lines will require removal by qualified practitioners in an operating theatre.

The role of non-medical prescribing in parenteral nutrition

Non-medical prescribing is defined by the Department of Health (2006) as prescribing by a practitioner (for example a dentist, nurse or pharmacist) responsible and accountable for the assessment of patients with undiagnosed or diagnosed conditions, and for making decisions about the clinical management of the patient, including prescribing.

From May 2006, qualified Nurse Independent Prescribers (formerly known as 'Extended Formulary Nurse Prescribers') have been able to prescribe any licensed medicine within the British National Formulary (BNF) for any medical condition within their competence, including some controlled drugs, whilst from the same date a new category of prescriber was created: the 'Pharmacist Independent Prescriber'. Pharmacist Independent Prescribers are able to prescribe any licensed medicine for any medical condition within their competence, with the exception of controlled drugs.

Non-medical prescribing offers many benefits for the patient, including increased choice, convenient access to medicines and more efficient service delivery. It also makes better use of nurses' and other health professionals' skills. Non-medical prescribing normally takes place within the context of a multidisciplinary team and is equally applicable in a hospital or community setting.

Pharmacists and nurses working within a hospital Nutrition Support Team with prescribing qualifications are able to prescribe PN as a supplementary prescriber. Supplementary prescribing is necessary because, although a bag of PN is licensed, the product becomes unlicensed once additional vitamins and electrolytes are added.

Non-medical prescribing has benefits for both the patient and Nutrition Support Team members particularly when there is no Nutrition Support Team clinician available, or the team works without the support of a clinician. Prior to the introduction of non-medical prescribing, it would have been necessary to request a prescription from a junior doctor with little or no PN prescribing experience, and often with very limited nutritional knowledge, that gave step-by-step details.

Conclusion

The decision to provide PN should not be considered an emergency. As this chapter shows, there are a number of risks associated with its provision. To minimise these risks, PN should be provided in conjunction with support and advice from a Nutrition Support Team, regular monitoring and a clear plan of therapy.

References

Bandregt, K., Soeters, P. (2005) *Nutritional Support in Clinical Nutrition*, Blackwell Science, London.

Burnham, P. (1999) Parenteral nutrition, in *Intravenous Therapy in Nursing Practice* (eds L. Dougherty, J. Lamb), Churchill Livingstone, Edinburgh.

Carlson, K.R. (1999) Correct utilisation and management of PICCs and midline catheters in the alternate care setting. *Journal of Intravenous Nursing* **22** (Supplement 6), S46–50.

Danks, L. (2006) Central venous catheters: A review of skin cleansing and dressings. *British Journal of Nursing* **15** (12), 650–4.

Department of Health (2001) Guidelines for preventing hospital acquired infections associated with the insertion and maintenance of central venous catheters. *Journal of Hospital Infection* **47** (Supplement), S47–67.

Department of Health (2006) *Improving Patient Access to Medicines: A Guide to Implementing Nurse and Pharmacist Independent Prescribing within the NHS in England*, DH, London.

Dougherty, L., Lister, S. (2008) *The Royal Marsden Manual of Clinical Nursing Procedures*, 7th edn, Blackwell Scientific, Oxford.

Farkas, J.C., Liu, N., Bleriot, J.P. *et al.* (1992) Single- versus triple-lumen central catheter-related sepsis: A prospective randomized study in a critically ill population. *American Journal of Medicine* **93** (3), 277–82.

Gabriel, J. (2000) What patients think of a PICC. *Journal of Vascular Access devices* **5** (4), 26–9.

Gabriel, J. (2001) PICC securement: Minimising potential complications. *Nursing Standard* **15** (43), 42–4.

Garland, J.S., Buck, R.K., Maloney, P. *et al.* (1995) Comparison of 10% povidone-iodine and 0.5% chlorhexidine gluconate for the prevention of peripheral intravenous catheter colonisation in neonates: A prospective trial. *Paediatric Infection Diseases Journal* **14** (6), 510–6.

Gillies, D., O'Riordan, L., Wallen, M. *et al.* (2004) Timing of intravenous administration set changes: A systematic review. *Infection Control and Hospital Epidemiology* **25** (3), 240–50.

Goetz, A.M., Wagener, M.M., Miller, J.M., Muder, R.R. (1998) Risk of infection due to central venous catheters: Effect of site of placement and catheter type. *Infection Control Hospital Epidemiology* **19** (11), 842–5.

Hamilton, H. (2000) *Total Parenteral Nutrition: A practical guide for nurses*, Churchill Livingstone, Edinburgh.

Hamilton, H. (2006) Complications associated with venous access devices (part 2). *Nursing Standard* **20** (27), 59–65.

Hardy, G., Sizer, T. (1999) A stable influence. *Nursing Times* (Nutrition Supplement) **95** (33), S61–67.

Hearnshaw, S.A., Thompson, N.P. (2007) Use of parenteral nutrition in hospitals in the north of England. *Journal of Human Nutrition & Dietetics* **20** (1), 14–23.

Johnson, B.H., Rypins, E.B. (1990) Single-lumen vs double-lumen catheters for total parenteral nutrition: A randomized, prospective trial. *Archives of Surgery* **125** (8), 990–2.

Maki, D.G., Ringer, M., Alvarado, C.J. (1991) Prospective randomised trial of providone-iodine, alcohol and chlorhexidine for prevention of infection associated with central venous and arterial catheters. *Lancet* **338** (8763), 339–42.

McCarthy, M.C., Shives, J.K., Robison, R.J., Broadie, T.A. (1987) Prospective evaluation of single and triple lumen catheters in total parenteral nutrition. *Journal of Parenteral Enteral Nutrition* **11** (3), 259–62.

Mimoz, O., Villeminey, S., Ragot, S. *et al.* (2007) Chlorhexidine-based anti-septic solution vs alcohol-based povidone-iodine for central venous catheter care. *Archives of Internal Medicine* **167** (19), 2066–72.

Murphy, A., Scott, A. (2000) Artificial nutritional support: What are the options? *Pharmaceutical Journal* **17** (6), 146–54.

National Institute for Health and Clinical Excellence (2003) *Infection Control: Prevention of healthcare associated infection in primary and community care, Clinical Guideline CG2,* NICE, London.

National Institute for Health and Clinical Excellence (2006) *Nutrition Support in Adults: Oral nutrition support, enteral tube feeding and parenteral nutrition, Clinical Guideline 32,* NICE, London.

Palmer, D., McFie, J. (2001) Venous access for parenteral nutrition, in *Artificial Nutrition Support in Clinical Practice,* 2nd edn (eds J. Payne-James, G. Grimble, Silk, D.B.A), Greenwich Medical Media, London.

Pemberton, L.B., Ross, V., Cuddy, P. *et al.* (1986) No difference between standard and antiseptic central venous catheters: A prospective randomised trial. *Archives of Surgery* **131** (9), 986–9.

Pennington, C.R. (1990) Review article: Towards safer parenteral nutrition. *Alimentary Pharmacology & Therapeutics* **4** (5), 427–41.

Pennington, C.R., Fawcett, H., McWhirter, J. *et al.* (1996) *Current Perspectives on Parenteral Nutrition in Adults. A report by a working party of the British Association for Parenteral and Enteral Nutrition,* BAPEN, Maidenhead.

Perucca, R. (2001) Obtaining vascular access, in *Intravenous Therapy in Clinical Practice,* 2nd edn (J. Terry, L. Baranowski, R.A. Lonsway, C. Hedrick), WB Saunders, Philadelphia.

Royal College of Nursing (2005) *Royal College of Nursing Standards for Infusion Therapy,* RCN IV Therapy Forum, London.

Russell, M.K., Andrews, M.R., Brewer, C.K. *et al.* (2002) Standards for specialized nutritional support: Adult hospitalised patients, ASPEN Board of Directors and the Task Force on Standards for Specialized Nutrition Support for Hospitalized Adult Patients. *Nutrition in Clinical Practice* **17**, 384–391.

Sains, K. (2005) Clinical nutrition: Using neutraceuticals in critical care. *Hospital Pharmacist* **12**, 14–16.

Schummer, W., Schummer, C., Schelenz, C. (2003) Case report: The malfunctioning implanted venous access device. *British Journal of Nursing* **12** (4), 210–14.

Shenkin, A. (1995) Adult micronutrient requirements, in *Artificial Nutrition Support in Clinical Practice* (eds J. Payne-James, G. Grimble, D. Silk), Edward Arnold, London.

Sheppard, K., LeDesma, M., Morris, N.L., O'Connor, K. (1999) A prospective study of two intravenous catheter securement techniques in a skilled nursing facility. *Journal of Intravenous Nursing* **22** (3), 151–6.

Soulsby, C., Weekes, L. (2004) Estimating nutritional requirements for adults, in *A Pocket Guide to Clinical Nutrition 2004,* (eds V. Todovoric, A. Micklewright), British Dietetic Association, London.

Springhouse Corporation (2002) *Intravenous Therapy Made Incredibly Easy,* Springhouse, Lippincott, Williams & Wilkins, Philadelphia.

Stacey, R.G.W., Filshie, J., Skewes, D. (1991) Percutaneous insertion of Hickman type catheters. *British Journal of Hospital Medicine* **46**, 396–8.

Thomas, B., Bishop, J. (eds) (2007) *Manual of Dietetic Practice*, 4th edn, Blackwell Publishing, Oxford.

Timmis, L. (1998) PICC of the bunch: Peripherally inserted central catheter. *Nursing Times* **94** (33), 70–3.

Todd, J. (1998) Peripherally inserted central catheters. *Professional Nurse* **13** (5), 297–302.

Van den Berghe, G., Wilmer, A., Hermans, G. *et al.* (2003) Intensive insulin therapy in the medical ICU. *New England Journal of Medicine* **354** (5), 449–61.

Veterans Affairs Total Parenteral Nutrition Cooperative Study Group (1991) Perioperative parenteral nutrition in surgical patients, *New England Journal of Medicine* **325** (8), 525–32.

Weinstein, S.M. (2001) *Plumers Principles and Practices of Intravenous therapy*, 7th edn, Lippincott, Williams & Wilkins, Philadelphia.

Wilson, J. (2001) *Preventing Infection Associated with Intravenous Therapy: Infection control in clinical practice*, 2nd edn, Bailliere Tindall, London.

Further reading

Austin, P., Stroud, M. (2007) *Prescribing Adult Intravenous Nutrition*, Pharmaceutical Press, London.

Chapter 7

Re-Feeding Syndrome

Helen Hitchings and Harriet Gordon

Introduction

The term 're-feeding syndrome' refers to a potentially fatal combination of severe fluid and electrolyte shifts, and related metabolic implications, which can occur when nutrition support is commenced in malnourished patients.

It is defined as 'the metabolic and physiological consequences of the depletion, repletion, compartmental shifts and interrelationships of the following: phosphate, potassium, magnesium, glucose metabolism, vitamin deficiency and fluid restriction' (Soloman & Kirby, 1990).

Re-feeding syndrome was initially reported in prisoners of war from Japanese concentration camps suffering extreme starvation at the end of the Second World War. When the prisoners were provided with adequate food upon liberation, vast numbers of prisoners began to show signs of cardiac dysfunction, oedema and neurological changes (Schnitker *et al.*, 1951). Earlier investigations into the effects of starvation in a group of previously healthy volunteers in the 1940s showed that after a period of severe food restriction some of the subjects experienced cardiac failure when normal intake was resumed: re-feeding syndrome (Soloman & Kirkby, 1990). Despite this evidence, in the twenty-first century, some surgeons and general physicians still have a poor level of understanding of re-feeding syndrome and its treatment (Hearing, 2004).

There is a more universal recognition of the development of re-feeding syndrome with the introduction of parenteral nutrition to malnourished patients but less recognition of its development with enteral feeding. Many patients at risk of re-feeding syndrome are treated on general wards and not in specialist nutrition units, especially those that are enterally fed. Therefore, to help prevent the development of re-feeding syndrome, awareness and understanding need to be increased to ensure that clinicians and nurses learn to recognise the signs of a patient at risk and avoid introducing over-aggressive nutrition support regimens too rapidly. It is therefore not too difficult to recognise why the National Institute of Health and Clinical Excellence (NICE; 2006) states that 'People at high risk of developing re-feeding problems should be cared for by healthcare professionals who are skilled and trained and have expert knowledge of nutritional requirements and nutritional support.'

To understand the process of re-feeding syndrome, it is first necessary to explore the effect of starvation on the body.

The process of starvation

As food intake decreases, there is less carbohydrate available for energy. This leads to a corresponding reduction in insulin concentration, and an increase in glucagon levels. The body begins to use fat and protein as alternative sources of energy.

During this process:

- Glycogen stores in the liver are rapidly converted to glucose, within the first 24 hours, and gluconeogenesis is activated, resulting in glucose synthesis from protein and fat breakdown products.
- Adipose tissue lipase is activated, releasing large amounts of fatty acids and glycerol. Free fatty acids and ketone bodies replace glucose as the major energy source.

During starvation, there is a loss of skeletal and cardiac muscle mass, owing to catabolism, which leads to an overall depletion in total body phosphate and other electrolytes. The intracellular electrolyte levels drop, often despite a relatively normal blood serum level. This is seen particularly with phosphate levels. If the patient is suffering from vomiting or diarrhoea, there is an additional loss of phosphate, magnesium and potassium, compounding the problem.

When carbohydrate is re-introduced, there is a switch from fat to carbohydrate metabolism, and there is a change from catabolism to stimulation of anabolic protein synthesis. Insulin levels rise, and there is a rapid intracellular uptake of electrolytes (phosphate, potassium and magnesium), glucose and water. As a consequence, the blood serum levels of electrolytes can drop profoundly, particularly phosphate, magnesium, potassium and calcium. During this stage, fluid retention may be noted. These effects are usually seen maximally at day three of commencing carbohydrate intake.

Incidence of re-feeding syndrome

Re-feeding syndrome can occur in anyone recommencing nutritional intake. Enterally fed patients can be as much at risk as those fed parenterally (Lauts, 2005; Marinella, 2004). Although less common, it can also occur in patients fed orally (Fung & Rimmer, 2005).

In the United Kingdom, patients found to be at particular risk include:

- those who have not been fed for more than seven days (e.g. post-surgical patients)
- chronic alcoholics
- chronic antacid users
- chronic diuretic users
- oncology patients, including those having chemotherapy
- those suffering from kwashiorkor or marasmus
- those with chronic malnutrition (e.g. patients with dysphagia following a stroke)
- those with anorexia nervosa
- those who have had anti-obesity surgery
- those with hyperglycaemia
- diabetics.
  (Cumming *et al.*, 1987; Holroyde *et al.*, 1977; Mason, 1998)

A study by Kagansky *et al.* (2005) found that approximately 14% of 2307 older patients examined had hypophosphataemia. They found that patients in the hypophosphataemic group had significantly more weight loss, lower albumin levels, more sepsis and received three times more glucose containing infusions and two times more food supplementations compared with the non-hypophosphataemic group. Patients in the hypophosphataemic group also had a significantly longer hospital stay and a reduced long-term survival, with a threefold increase in mortality rates.

NICE (2006) states that patients should be assessed for their risk of re-feeding syndrome and class risk using the following guide:

The patient is considered to be at **moderate risk** if they have one or more of the following:

- a body mass index (BMI) of less than 18.5 kg/m^2
- unintentional weight loss greater than 10% within the previous three to six months
- very little intake for longer than five days.

The patient is considered to be at **high risk** if they have one or more of the following:

- a BMI of less than 16 kg/m^2
- unintentional weight loss greater than 15% within the previous three to six months
- very little nutritional intake for longer than 10 days
- low levels of potassium, phosphate or magnesium prior to feeding.

They are also considered to be at high risk if they have two or more of the following:

- a BMI of less than 18.5 kg/m^2
- unintentional weight loss greater than 10% within the previous three to six months
- very little nutritional intake for longer than five days
- a history of alcohol abuse
- regularly takes insulin, antacids or diuretics
- recent chemotherapy treatment.

The patient is considered to be at **severely high risk** if they have one or more of the following:

- a BMI of less than 14 kg/m^2
- negligible intake for longer than 15 days.

Impact on the patient

The syndrome is potentially fatal and may well go unrecognised. It is more common in the elderly, probably because they tend to have significant comorbidity. Oncology patients having nutrition support have an incidence as high as 25% (Gonzalez *et al.*, 1996).

Starvation carries severe cardiorespiratory effects, with a loss of cardiac muscle mass, resulting in cardiac failure, and loss of skeletal and respiratory muscle, resulting in respiratory deficiency.

With the electrolyte shifts that occur as carbohydrate is re-introduced (as the patient receives nutrition), the effects of re-feeding are multiplied on an already compromised cardiovascular system.

The consequences of re-feeding syndrome include:

- hypophosphataemia
- hypomagnesaemia
- hypokalaemia
- altered glucose metabolism
- fluid-balance abnormalities
- vitamin deficiency.

Hypophosphataemia

Most phosphorus in the body (85%) is present in the form of hydroxy-apatite in the bone. The remaining 15% is mainly as phosphates or esters, and is a constituent of substances such as phospholipids, which are a major constituent of most biological membranes. It is present in all cells of the body, being an essential component of DNA and RNA. Phosphate is essential for phosphorylation, which is required to convert adenosine diphosphate (ADP) and adenosine monophosphate to adenosine triphosphate (ATP), which is required for the release of energy. It is also crucial in glycolysis. Phosphate concentration is controlled by calcium concentration, parathyroid hormone, vitamin D and renal function. Nutritionally depleted patients have a higher phosphate requirement and are at risk of clinically significant hypophosphataemia.

Those likely to have a pre-existing phosphate depletion are people who have:

- taken phosphate-binding antacids
- experienced gastrointestinal losses from diarrhoea and vomiting
- had an increased cellular uptake from liver failure, alcoholism, sepsis
- a vitamin D deficiency
- hyperparathyroidism, giving increased renal excretion
- become critically ill with an alkalosis
- X-linked familial hypophosphataemia
- diabetic ketoacidosis
- used some types of diuretic drugs.

The kidney is the major site for regulating the amount of phosphorus retained in the body. Normal serum phosphate levels are in the region of 0.78 to 1.53 mmol/l. The consequences of hypophosphataemia (levels less than 0.3 mmol/l) include:

- arrhythmias
- cardiac failure
- respiratory failure
- rhabdomyolysis
- haematological   abnormalities,   in   particular   white-cell
  dysfunction
- convulsions
- coma
- death.

Treatment for hypophosphataemia of levels of less than 0.5 mmol/l may be done safely with a Phosphates Polyfusor infusion (Terlevich *et al.*, 2003), although in some patients there is concern about the sodium content of the Phosphates Polyfusor. There are other products available which can be administered intravenously, such as monobasic potassium phosphate. For those patients receiving enteral nutrition, supplements such as Phosphate Sandoz can be used. However, patients should be made aware that diarrhoea is a common side effect. Any phosphate supplementation can cause hypocalcaemia, and so it is essential to closely monitor plasma concentrations of calcium, phosphate, potassium and other electrolytes whilst phosphate replacement is undertaken.

Hypokalaemia

Potassium is the major intracellular cation and primary intracellular buffer, playing a fundamental role in acid-base regulation, fluid balance, muscle contraction and nerve conduction. It maintains the neuromuscular electrical potential and is important in acid-base balance (with hydrogen ions) and osmotic pressure (with sodium). Potassium is essential for the function of the Na-K-ATPase pump, which uptakes solutes into cells, including glucose. Abnormalities of potassium concentration affect cardiac excitability and hypo- or hyperkalaemia can lead to cardiac arrhythmias.

Excretion is regulated by the kidney, with only minimal amounts lost in sweat and faeces.

Normal potassium levels are about 3.6–5.1 mmol/l.

Those at risk of hypokalaemia include:

- patients on diuretics, unless potassium sparing
- patients with increased gastrointestinal losses (e.g. diarrhoea and vomiting, surgical patients with fistulae, wound drains, nasogastric aspirates)

- patients with a metabolic alkalosis
- patients with an increased cellular uptake of potassium (e.g. beta-2 agonists, insulin, acute alkalosis)
- patients with low magnesium levels (which may contribute to hypokalaemia; in patients who have a persistent hypokalaemia, regular monitoring of magnesium levels is recommended)
- patients with diabetic ketoacidosis.

Potassium depletion may also be a consequence of excessive sodium intake.

The consequences of hypokalaemia include:

- rhabdomyolysis
- respiratory depression
- paralytic ileus
- glucose intolerance
- arrhythmias, cardiac arrest.

In severe hypokalaemia (<2.5 mmol/l – or symptomatic) correction should be by careful intravenous infusion. Potassium salts are irritants and can cause phlebitis if administered through smaller veins. A maximum concentration of 40 mmol/l (3 g/l) potassium may be given by peripheral infusion; higher concentrations should be administered via a central line.

The usual maximum recommended rate of infusion is 10 mmol/hr, although higher rates (for example 20 mmol/hr) may be given with electrocardiographic (ECG) monitoring. Refer to local guidelines.

Patients able to tolerate oral or enteral therapy and those with less severe hypokalaemia (2.5–3.5 mmol/l or asymptomatic) may be treated with potassium effervescent tablets. However, nausea and vomiting are common side effects.

IV correction should be used if the patient has diarrhoea or a high-output stoma.

The input of a pharmacist is essential to ensure that the patient is not on any medication that could cause a rise in plasma potassium concentration. It is also essential to continue to monitor the effect of any supplementation, by repeating blood biochemistry checks during and immediately after the administration of potassium.

Hypomagnesaemia

Magnesium is the second most abundant mineral in the human body, about half of which is present in the skeleton, with the remainder mostly being within body cells. Magnesium is primarily an intracellular electrolyte critical in metabolic processes, being involved with aerobic and anaerobic energy generation. It is an essential constituent for many enzymes, particularly those involved in energy generation, including ATP-dependent cation transport (sodium and calcium). It interacts with calcium to affect the neuromuscular excitability and membrane potentials. As well as playing a vital role in skeletal development, it is essential for protein synthesis, muscle contraction and neurotransmission. Hypomagnesaemia is associated with other electrolyte deficiencies, including hypokalaemia and hypophosphataemia.

Magnesium is secreted in large amounts in gastrointestinal fluid.

The kidney plays a key role in magnesium homeostasis.

Those at risk include:

- patients with severe diarrhoea, or losses through stomas or fistulas
- patients with pancreatitis
- patients with hyper- or hypoparathyroidism
- patients with sepsis.

Consequences of hypomagnesaemia include:

- parasthesiae
- seizures
- cardiac arrhythmias
- hypertension.

Normal magnesium levels are approximately 0.74–1.03 mmol/l.

Mild hypomagnesaemia (>0.5 mmol/l) may be treated orally if the patient is able to tolerate oral or enteral therapy. However, magnesium salts are not well absorbed from the gastrointestinal tract.

Treatment is more effective if given intravenously with magnesium sulphate as an infusion, if the level is less than 0.5 mmol/l, or if the patient is receiving intravenous therapy only.

Hypocalcaemia

Calcium is the most abundant mineral in the body, with 99% of this mineral found within the skeleton. Serum calcium can be bound to proteins, complexes with other ions or remain as free ions. The functions of calcium include maintaining structure in the bones and the regulation of membrane potentials, a vital role affecting membrane transport and stability. It acts as a co-factor for certain enzymes and influences functions such as muscle contraction and nerve transmission. It also has a role to play as a co-factor for coagulation.

As serum calcium is affected by albumin levels, it can be useful to use a 'corrected calcium' level.

Corrected calcium levels for low albumin are calculated using one of the following equations:

$$\text{serum calcium (mmol/l)} + \frac{(40 - \text{albumin})}{40}$$

An alternative and possibly more accurate equation is:

$$\text{serum calcium (mmol/l)} + [(40 - \text{albumin}) \times 0.02]$$

To be even more accurate, the effect of serum protein should also be incorporated changing the equation to:

$$\text{serum calcium (mmol/l)} + [(72 - \text{protein}) \times 0.02]$$

This final corrected calcium value should be added to that obtained from the correction for low albumin (the second calculation), and the average of the two levels obtained, calculated to two decimal places (Thomas & Bishop, 2007).

Those at risk of a reduced calcium level include:

- renal-failure patients
- those with hyperparathyroidism, hypomagnesaemia, hyperphosphataemia
- those with pancreatitis
- those with chronic diarrhoea.

Clinically, the consequences include:

- muscle cramps
- parasthesiae
- tetany
- arrhythmias
- convulsions.

Treatment is by administration of calcium gluconate 10% injection as a slow IV injection or diluted for administration by IV infusion.

Thiamine (vitamin B1) deficiency

Starvation is associated with several vitamin deficiencies, including thiamine.

Thiamine is an essential co-factor for a variety of enzyme activities involved in carbohydrate metabolism, and is also required for the normal functioning of the nervous system.

As with most water-soluble vitamins, very little free thiamine is stored in the tissues. If commencing feeding in an already thiamine-depleted patient, further depletion will occur, as carbohydrate ingestion is associated with an increased cellular uptake of thiamine. This could result in a clinical presentation of deficiency, the Wernicke–Korsakov syndrome which is an acute neurological abnormality, characterised by:

- Wernicke's encephalopathy (confusion, ataxia, coma, ocular disturbances)
- Korsakov's syndrome (short-term memory loss, confabulation).

The biological half life of thiamine is approximately 10 to 20 days. Experimental depletion of thiamine has shown that biochemical signs of deficiency can be observed within 10 days, and physiological changes within 28 days. Marginal deficiency can develop rapidly, particularly in alcoholics, who may have low liver stores. Symptoms of subclinical deficiency can include headaches, tiredness, anorexia and muscle wasting.

Body fluid homeostasis

Re-feeding syndrome can cause disturbances in the body's fluid distribution, resulting in either dehydration or fluid overload. If untreated, the patients could develop:

- cardiac failure
- hypotension
- pre-renal failure
- sudden death.

Carbohydrate feeding can lead to a reduction in sodium and water excretion. This together with the movement of sodium from the intracellular space to the extracellular space with increased ATP production will expand the extracellular fluid compartment, precipitating weight gain manifesting as oedema or ascites, particularly if sodium intake is increased (Crook *et al.*, 2002).

Summary of electrolyte disturbances

Patients at risk of electrolyte disturbances include:

- the critically ill
- those with alkalosis
- those with sepsis
- those with excess GI losses
- those with other electrolyte disturbances.

The consequences of electrolyte disturbances include:

- arrhythmias, so that ECG monitoring is advisable
- neuromuscular disturbances with symptoms of cramps and paraesthesiae, and progressing to cardiorespiratory depression, convulsions and death.

Reducing the risk of re-feeding syndrome

Education of hospital staff

Many patients are potentially at risk of re-feeding; however, clearly not all will manifest the syndrome. The Nutrition Support Team is in an ideal position to provide education and support for ward staff (Landau-West *et al.*, 1993). However, it is important to educate all healthcare professionals about the risks of re-feeding syndrome, the monitoring required and the step-by-step approach to re-introducing feeding in the malnourished patient.

Identify those at risk

Water-soluble vitamins

Give a high-dose, water-soluble vitamin supplement, to include thiamine, for a few days (for example Pabrinex infusion, one pair of ampoules daily for three days) to those at high risk. This may be started a few days before any nutrition is commenced, and in high-risk patients should be commenced at least 30 minutes prior to initiating any feeding. Staff should be made aware that anaphylaxis has been reported after repeated Pabrinex infusion.

Where tolerated, oral thiamine can and should be given for the first 10 days of feeding, 200–300 mg daily, together with one or two tablets of Vitamin B Compound strong three times daily, and a balanced multivitamin/trace-element supplement once daily until full feeding is established (National Institute for Health and Clinical Excellence, 2006).

Electrolyte monitoring

Electrolyte levels should be measured to establish a baseline prior to commencing any nutrition support. However, it is not necessary to correct any abnormal low plasma levels prior to starting feeding (National Institute for Health and Clinical Excellence, 2006). It is more important to monitor changes that occur on commencing feeding; this should include noting sodium, potassium, calcium, magnesium and phosphate levels. Then they need to be monitored daily for the first week. Prior to commencing feeding, many patients have normal blood biochemistry in the starved state, owing to changes in renal excretion. However, this should not give a false sense of security. Levels are likely to fall on commencing feeding. It is essential to monitor and correct these electrolyte levels in the early stages of feeding. If additional supplementation of electrolytes is required, it may be necessary to wait until distribution has been achieved in the body before re-checking the levels; for example, after administering a Phosphates Polyfusor, it would be wise to wait for six hours before re-checking phosphate levels to obtain an accurate result.

Electrolyte levels may need to be corrected intravenously for phosphate (give 50 mmol phosphate over 24 hours), potassium and magnesium as it may not be possible to achieve adequate levels orally.

Electrocardiographic monitoring

Tachycardia is often the first indication of the development of life-threatening arrhythmias. If this occurs, ECG monitoring is essential for the monitoring of further disturbances.

Start feeding slowly

Any patient who has received very little nutritional intake for longer than five days is at some risk of re-feeding problems. Nutrition for these patients should be started at no more than 50% of requirements for the first 48 hours. If close biochemical and clinical monitoring reveals no re-feeding problems, nutrition can be increased to meet full requirements.

Patients assessed as being at high risk of re-feeding syndrome should start feeding at low levels of protein and energy, but with adequate provision of group B vitamins, including thiamine, and all other vitamins, minerals and trace elements. This may mean starting at energy levels as low as 10 kcal/kg. With close monitoring and correction of abnormal electrolyte levels, nutrition can be increased towards meeting full requirements by seven days.

In patients assessed as being at severe risk of re-feeding problems, nutrition should be started at 5 kcal/kg. Continual cardiac monitoring is recommended in this group of patients (National Institute for Health and Clinical Excellence, 2006), and in any other patients who have, or develop, cardiac arrhythmias.

Providing such low levels of nutrition initially is very likely to result in suboptimal fluid levels. Therefore, the medical team will need to be made aware of the need to supply additional fluids. Calories should be increased slowly, over the following 10 days. During this period, fluid-balance and electrolyte levels will need careful monitoring.

The patient will need to be monitored for:

- electrolyte abnormalities in the first few days, maximal at day three
- cardiac complications, which may manifest over the first week
- neurological features (tremor, seizures, coma) after that (Crook *et al.*, 2001).

It is perhaps natural to want to provide sufficient or even excessive nutritional intakes to those who are the most malnourished. However, owing to the risks of re-feeding syndrome, it is essential to provide less in terms of energy initially then and, with close and thorough monitoring, gradually increase this to meet perceived requirements. Maintain regular contact with your Nutrition Support Team or ward dietitian to ensure the appropriate support and advice is obtained.

Ward checklist for re-feeding syndrome

1. Identify patients at risk of re-feeding
   - patients who have not been fed for longer than seven days
   - alcoholics
   - antacid users
   - diuretic users
   - oncology patients
   - patients with chronic malnutrition, e.g. stroke
   - patients with anorexia nervosa

    ○   those who have had anti-obesity surgery
    ○   patients with hyperglycaemia
    ○   diabetics

2. Monitor electrolytes before and during first 10 days of feeding, particularly sodium, magnesium, phosphate and calcium, and correct as required.
3. Give water-soluble vitamins, e.g. Pabrinex, one pair ampoules for three days, commence before feeding starts.
4. Monitor with an ECG if indicated.
5. Start feeding slowly, dependent upon risk of re-feeding problems, and increase slowly over 10 days, provided there are no adverse consequences.

Conclusion

Re-feeding syndrome is a condition which often goes unrecognised but if left untreated could have fatal consequences for the malnourished patient when nutrition is first re-introduced. With increased awareness and careful monitoring, it is possible to minimise the risks caused by electrolyte shifts and provide treatment which will enhance the metabolism of carbohydrate in the early stages of nutrition support.

References

Crook, M.A., Hally, V., Panteli, J.V. (2001) The importance of the refeeding syndrome. *Nutrition* **17**, 632–7.

Crook, M., Panteli, J., Horn, V. (2002) *Guidelines for the prevention and management of the refeeding syndrome*, University Hospital Lewisham NHS Trust, London.

Cumming, A.D., Farquar, J.R., Bouchier, I.A.D. (1987) Refeeding hypophosphataemia in anorexia nervosa and alcoholism. *British Medical Journal* **295**, 490–1.

Fung, A.T., Rimmer, J. (2005) Hypophosphataemia secondary to oral refeeding syndrome in a patient with long-term alcohol misuse. *Medical Journal of Australia* **183** (6), 324–6.

Gonzalez, A.G., Fajardo-Rodriguez, A., Gonzalez-Figueroa, E. (1996) The incidence of the refeeding syndrome in cancer patients who receive artificial nutritional treatment. *Nutrición Hospitalaria* (English abstract) **11**, 98.

Hearing, S.D. (2004) Refeeding syndrome: Is underdiagnosed and undertreated, but treatable. *British Medical Journal* **328**, 908–9.

Holroyde, C.P., Myers, R.N., Smink, R.D. *et al.* (1977) Metabolic response to total parenteral nutrition in cancer patients. *Cancer Research* **37**, 3109–14.

Kagansky, N., Levy, S., Koren-Morag, N. *et al.* (2005) Hypophosphataemia in old patients is associated with the refeeding syndrome and reduced survival. *Journal of Internal Medicine* **257** (5), 461–8.

Landau-West, D., Kohl, D., Pasulka, P. (1993) Team management of eating disorders. *Nutrition in Clinical Practice* **8**, 220.

Lauts, N.M. (2005) Management of the patient with refeeding syndrome. *Journal of Infusion Nursing* **28** (5), 337–42.

Marinella, M.A. (2004) Refeeding syndrome: Implications for the inpatient rehabilitation unit. *American Journal of Physical Medicine & Rehabilitation/ Association of Academic Physiatrists* **83** (1), 65–8.

Mason, E.E. (1998) Starvation injury after gastric reduction for obesity. *World Journal of Surgery* **22** (9), 1002–7.

National Institute for Health and Clinical Excellence (2006) *Nutrition Support in Adults: Oral nutrition support, enteral tube feeding and parenteral nutrition, Clinical Guideline 32*, NICE, London.

Schnitker, M.A., Mattman, P.E., Bliss, T.L. (1951) A clinical study of malnutrition in Japanese prisoners of war. *Annals of Internal Medicine* **35**, 69–96.

Soloman, S.M., Kirby, D.F. (1990) The refeeding syndrome: A review. *Journal of Parenteral and Enteral Nutrition* **14**, 90–7.

Terlevich, A., Hearing, S.D., Woltersdorf, W.W. *et al.* (2003) Refeeding syndrome: Effective and safe treatment with 'phosphates polyfusor'. *Alimentary Pharmacology and Therapeutics* **17**, 1325–9.

Thomas, B., Bishop, J. (eds) (2007) *Manual of Dietetic Practice*, 4th edn, Blackwell Publishing, Oxford.

Chapter 8

Ethics and Commitment to Feed

Carolyn Best

Introduction

Dehydration, weight loss and malnutrition are likely outcomes for a patient who has an irretrievable decline in oral intake. Persisting with an oral diet when swallowing difficulties develop may put the patient at risk of developing aspiration pneumonia. The provision of nutrition support or artificial nutrition in the form of nasogastric or gastrostomy tube feeding may overcome some of these difficulties and provide a regular and appropriate level of nutrition and fluid, but it cannot be expected to restore the patient's level of function or consciousness. Patients who are seriously ill or in the terminal phase of their illness do not respond to the administration of nutrition support in the same way as patients who have the potential for recovery (Smith & Andrews, 2000). The decision to proceed with nutrition support should be based on the principles that it will benefit the patient by restoring or maintaining health, maximising benefit and minimising harm (British Medical Association, 2002).

There will be circumstances in which the provision of nutrition support is not clinically indicated or where risks of trying to provide nutrition outweigh the potential benefits, for example advanced dementia (see below). The prolongation of life will usually be in the best interests of a patient, provided that the treatment is not excessively burdensome or disproportionate to the expected benefits (National Institute for Health and Clinical Excellence, 2006). It is clear that for anyone contemplating the provision of nutrition support a number of ethical and legal decisions need to be considered.

The introduction of nutrition support was originally intended to offer support until normal digestive functioning (or swallowing ability) was restored (Macfie, 2001), but technological advances and higher expectations of the right to treatment have led to the provision of nutrition support for many groups of patients who have lost the ability to maintain their nutritional intake regardless of their potential for recovery or level of functionality, ensuring the survival of increasing numbers of patients with severe physical or cognitive impairment.

Owing to an unrealistic or inaccurate expectation of what nutrition support can accomplish (Angus & Burakoff, 2003), healthcare professionals may feel they have an obligation to provide nutrition support as the technology is available, but consideration should be given to why the treatment is being proposed and whether it is deemed to be in the best interests of the patient. It could be argued that the answer is no, if the intervention will not improve the quality of the patient's life.

There is a belief that dehydration is uncomfortable and that as food and drink are basic necessities of life it is unethical to allow someone to starve to death. The response to a patient's inability to eat or drink will depend upon the aim of care. If the patient is in an advanced stage of their illness, it is normal to see a reduction in eating and drinking. It may not be that the patient is refusing or is unable to eat or drink but that they are dying and therefore do not wish to do so (Lennard-Jones, 1999).

It is therefore quite clear that decision-making in relation to the provision or withholding of nutrition support must be handled carefully. To minimise misunderstanding and disagreements, open and frank discussions will be required during any decision-making process as this aspect of care can evoke emotive responses, and decisions to provide or withhold nutrition support may cause upset for family and healthcare professionals involved in the patient's care.

To assist decision-making in these circumstances the Council of the British Association for Parenteral and Enteral Nutrition issued a report entitled *Ethical and Legal Aspects of Clinical Hydration and Nutritional Support* (Lennard-Jones, 1998) in which it makes a number of recommendations, including:

- A patient who can swallow and expresses a desire or willingness to drink or eat should be encouraged and assisted to do so and provided with appropriate fluid and nutrients as part of their basic care.
- If the plan is to provide compassionate care for relief of symptoms during the terminal phase of illness, oral fluid and food should be given according to the patient's wishes and ability to swallow;

Loan Receipt
Liverpool John Moores University
Library Services

Borrower Name: Dove,Chloe
Borrower ID: *********9118

Promoting physical activity :
31111013327315
Due Date: 06/02/2015 23:59

Nutrition :
31111012643258
Due Date: 06/02/2015 23:59

Total Items: 2
16/01/2015 16:05

Please keep your receipt in case of
dispute.

fluid given through a tube should only be given if it is needed to relieve thirst.
- Fluid given via a tube is regarded in law as a medical treatment.

Benefits vs burden

If nutrition support extends a period of life but not its quality, it may provide comfort to a relative or healthcare professional, who may feel that in insisting that nutrition support is provided they will have done 'something to help', but we need to consider the issue from the patient's perspective. Will this decision be of benefit to them? Whilst a healthcare professional has a duty to prolong life, they do not have a duty to inappropriately prolong dying. The British Medical Association (BMA; 2002) states that if nutrition support and hydration provide the patient with some benefit, they should be provided. Once the decision is made to provide nutrition support, another major dilemma arises when the treatment stops providing benefit to the patient or becomes harmful. Often, the decision to withdraw nutrition support can be more difficult than making the decision to provide it.

Informed consent

To be valid, informed consent must be given by a mentally competent patient voluntarily and without duress or fraud (Dimond, 2005). For consent to be informed, the patient must be provided with sufficient information regarding the benefits and risks of the proposed treatment, any risks of non-treatment and be made aware of any possible alternative treatments. The Nursing and Midwifery Council (NMC; 2004) states that all patients have the right to receive information regarding their condition and that the information should be accurate, truthful and given in such a way as to make it easily understood. If the patient is not offered as much information as they reasonably need to make their decision, and in a form that they can understand, their consent may not be valid (Department of Health, 2001a).

The provision of nutrition via a feeding tube is considered to be medical treatment that can be refused, withheld or withdrawn (Lennard-Jones, 1999). Therefore, consent must be given prior to commencing all forms of nutrition support. In law, there is no specific requirement that consent should be given in any particular way (Dimond, 2005). It makes no difference whether people sign a form to indicate their consent or give consent orally or even non-verbally, for example by holding out an arm for blood pressure to be taken (Department of Health, 2001b).

It is good practice to seek written consent if treatment is complex or involves significant risks or side effects, such as the insertion of a percutaneous endoscopic gastrostomy (PEG) tube or central catheter. However, a signature on a consent form does not, in itself, prove the consent is valid and voluntary. A consent form is only a record of the patient's decision, and shows that discussions have taken place regarding the risks and benefits of the proposed procedure or treatment. It is not proof that genuine consent has been given (Dimond, 2005).

Seeking consent should be seen as a *process*, not a one-off event. When seeking a person's consent to treatment or care, you should make sure that they are given the time and support they need to make their decision. People who have given consent to a particular intervention are entitled to change their minds and withdraw their consent at any point if they have the capacity to do so (Department of Health, 2001b).

Decision-making in the competent patient

In order for consent to be valid in law, the patient must be capable of making that decision. Adult patients are presumed to have the capacity to make a decision regarding their care unless it is established that they lack capacity to do so (Department of Health, 2005a). Assessment of competence is based on the ability to demonstrate adequate thought processes necessary to reach a decision (Lennard-Jones, 1998).

If, after discussion of treatment options, a competent patient refuses treatment, the decision must be respected, even if a refusal of treatment may ultimately lead to their death. Indeed, the Mental Capacity Act (Department of Health, 2005a) states that a person is not to be treated as unable to make a decision merely because he makes an unwise decision. Where this occurs, the decision should be clearly documented in the patient's notes. If the patient has already signed a consent form, but then changes their mind, documentation to this effect should be recorded on the previously signed consent form. The patient is still free to change their mind and accept treatment at a later date if they wish to do so but should be advised of the effects of that delay (Department of Health, 2001a). A competent adult's decision to refuse treatment should not be overridden by healthcare profession-

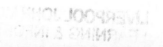

als. However, it is important that the patient is deemed to be mentally competent.

Some patients do not wish to exercise their right of choice and prefer to leave the decisions to those who care for them. This may imply acceptance of the treatment recommended (implied consent). Implied consent is not, however, supported in law (Dimond, 2005). The problem with implied consent is that it is not always clear that the patient is agreeing to the treatment recommended. Unless communication from the health professional is clear, the patient may be giving non-verbal consent for what they understand to be the treatment but which, without clarification of understanding, may be something quite different. To limit misunderstanding, the health professional should communicate clearly and encourage the patient, where possible, to participate in the decision-making process.

It is ethically and legally wrong for a carer to underestimate the capacity of a patient in order to achieve what the carer believes to be in the patient's best interests.

If a person has the capacity to consent to treatment for which written consent is usual but cannot write or is physically unable to sign a form, a record that the person has given oral or non-verbal consent should be made in their notes or on the consent form.

Decision-making in the non-competent patient

The terms 'non-competent' and 'lacks capacity' refer to the inability of an individual to make a particular decision or take a particular action for themselves at the time the decision or action needs to be taken (Department of Health, 2005a). The Mental Capacity Act 2005 (Department of Health, 2005a) provides a statutory framework to empower and protect these people who are potentially vulnerable and clearly identifies who can take decisions on the patient's behalf, in which situations and how they should go about this.

Adequate consultation with the patient is necessary when there is a need to change, stop or start a treatment. Unfortunately for some patients, by the time they require nutrition support, they may be unable to exercise their right to consent, owing to fluctuating levels of comprehension or a loss of capacity to assess physical harm against the presumed benefits of the proposed treatment.

When assessing the capacity of the patient, it is imperative to assess whether the loss of capacity is temporary or is likely to be permanent. The person who lacks capacity to make a decision for themselves at a particular time may be in a position to make that decision at a later date if:

- they have an illness or condition that means their capacity changes as they recover, or
- because at the time the decision needs to be made their level of consciousness is compromised, e.g. because of an accident or when the patient is under an anaesthetic (Department of Health, 2005a).

A person is not to be treated as unable to make a decision unless all practicable steps to help them to do so have been taken without success (Department of Health, 2005a). Therefore, where there are fluctuating levels of comprehension attempts should be made to discuss treatment options with the patient at a time when their comprehension is clear. Where this proves difficult or where there is uncertainty as to the patient's ability to make decisions, a test to assess for a patient's level of competence should be used (Department of Health, 2005a).

A lack of capacity does not diminish the right of the patient to receive or refuse treatment but rather places the onus on healthcare professionals to act in their best interests.

Under English Law, a relative does not have the right to make a decision on behalf of a patient (Dimond, 2005) unless they have a lasting power of attorney, but they could play an instrumental part by providing valuable information regarding the patient's beliefs and wishes.

In the case of an adult patient who lacks capacity, the doctor in charge of that patient's care is responsible in law for any decision to withhold, withdraw or commence a medical treatment (Lennard-Jones, 1998). At all times, decisions made on behalf of the patient should be in the patient's best interests. Any previously expressed views regarding the level and type of treatment the patient would wish to receive must be considered, especially if there is a written record or advanced directive.

Best interests

In some situations, in order to protect the vulnerable adult, it may be necessary to take decisions on their behalf. It is important that those making the decision are acting in the best interests of the individual.

In determining whether the provision of a treatment is in a person's best interests, the following factors should be considered:

- What actions are necessary to promote the individual's health or well-being or to prevent a deterioration in their quality of life?
- Their capacity to make a decision at the time the decision is needed. If the patient lacks capacity at that particular time, is their ability to make a decision likely to return at some point in the future and when is that likely to be?
- The need to encourage the person to participate as fully as possible in anything done for them and any decision affecting them.
- Whether the intervention is necessary.
- If intervention is necessary, seek to ensure that it is as limited as possible to maintain safety.
- That any decision made is within the confines of the law.
- Their known wishes and feelings and the factors they would consider if they were able to do so.
- That the expressed wishes of the person without capacity were not made as the result of undue influence.
- Whether they had previously recorded their wishes in relation to a specified treatment in an advanced directive (or living will).
- The views of other people whom it is appropriate and practicable to consult about the person's wishes and feelings and what would be in their best interests (Department of Health, 2005b).

A decision to provide treatment should not be based on the person's age or appearance, or behaviour (Department of Health, 2005b). Where the decision relates to the provision of life-sustaining treatment, consideration of best interest must not be motivated by a desire to bring about their death. Decisions in such circumstances should never be made by an individual. The need for multidisciplinary discussion is essential during this process as deciding what is in the best interests of patients will vary.

Advanced directives

An advanced directive, or living will, involves the patient making decisions when competent regarding their wishes on future care and treatment should they become ill and are no longer able to communicate or lose the capacity to make an informed decision. In the United Kingdom, advanced directives are recognised in common law (Dimond, 2005).

An advanced directive allows an individual to:

- give their consent to particular forms of treatment
- refuse treatments: may be used in relation to life-sustaining treatments (e.g. resuscitation or nutrition support)
- appoint someone to make decisions on their behalf regarding their future care and treatment (lasting power of attorney).

An advanced directive is only valid if it is reviewed regularly to ensure it remains relevant. Providing that the advanced directive is 'clearly established and applicable to the circumstances' the patient is in, it is legally binding (Keown, 2003). Therefore, if a patient has made an advanced directive detailing their wishes regarding nutrition support, they must be followed (British Medical Association, 2002) regardless of whether or not it is deemed to be of most benefit to the patient. A healthcare professional who overrides the wishes of a competent patient or an advanced directive may be liable in law for battery (Keown, 2003).

Power of attorney

Under the Mental Capacity Act (Department of Health, 2005a), lasting power of attorney (LPA) replaces the enduring power of attorney (EPA) as the primary way of choosing a decision-maker to act on behalf of an individual should they lose their mental capacity (Dimond, 2007). As with the EPA, an LPA allows the decision-maker to make decisions in relation to property and affairs but also confers the additional power of decision-making in relation to personal welfare, including healthcare.

Percutaneous endoscopic gastrostomy feeding in advanced dementia

Patients with advanced dementia frequently develop swallowing problems, eating difficulties or an indifference to food (Morris *et al.*, 1989; Young-In, 2001) leading to a reduction in nutritional intake, weight loss and an increased risk of aspiration.

When these circumstances arise, family members or healthcare professionals may press to find alternative methods of providing fluid and nutrition. However, the provision of nutrition support may not be the most appropriate course of action to take. The insertion of a feeding tube is not without risk. Indeed, Sanders *et al.* (2000) suggest that patients with advanced dementia have a higher rate of mortality when compared to patients without dementia following the insertion of a PEG tube. They report mortality rates at one month post PEG insertion of 54% in patients with dementia compared to 28% in non-dementia patients and 90% at one year compared to 63%. Finucane *et al.* (1999) take this one step further by stating that there are no direct data to support tube feeding in patients with dementia. Hoffer (2006) notes that severely demented patients fail to benefit from tube feeding for two reasons: they lack the potential for physical or neurological rehabilitation and they are not starving. He argues that as the individual progresses into the advanced stage of dementia they have a low metabolic rate. This is attributed to muscle wasting that has diminished lean body mass and to a brain that has atrophied. He goes on to state that although people with advanced dementia may be thin and eat less food they are in a state of physiological homeostasis.

This is supported by the evidence provided in the General Medical Council (GMC) appeal to the *Burke* case – R (*Leslie Burke*) vs *GMC* [2004] EWHC 1879 (Admin) – during which the GMC argued nutrition support and hydration should be withheld in patients with advanced dementia as no overt distress is displayed through lack of fluid or nutrients. Li (2002) suggests that PEG feeding may actually increase discomfort in advanced dementia as it takes away the pleasure of tasting food and the moistening of the oral cavity as fluid is consumed.

Finucane *et al.* (1999) state that patients who were hand-fed showed a more favourable survival rate compared to those who had received PEG and had similar survival rates to non-demented patients. In studies questioning competent individuals (Hoefler, 2000; McNamara & Kennedy, 2001), many people indicated that they would not wish to receive nutrition support if they developed advanced dementia.

In view of these findings, it would seem sensible to suggest that for the patient with advanced dementia initiatives to prolong oral intake should be explored, for example:

- providing finger foods
- altering flavours or consistencies of food
- offering food that is presented well and in appropriate portions

- checking dentures fit correctly
- treating the onset of depression
- providing an increased level of assistance with eating when necessary
- providing families and carers with a balanced view of likely outcomes when considering the provision of nutrition support versus continued oral feeding.

Persistent vegetative state

The condition of persistent vegetative state (PVS) is on the border between coma and awareness. A person in a PVS has no awareness of self or their environment and is incapable of interacting with others (Lennard-Jones, 1998). A vegetative state may be temporary or permanent. Patients in the vegetative state are unable to give consent, both literally and legally (in terms of their mental capacity). Therefore, when considering treatments, the principle of best interest must be used.

In these patients, the provision of enteral feeding may keep them alive for many years. Where consideration is given to the withdrawal of feeding, an application to the court should be made regarding the legality of such an action. In the case of Anthony Bland (*Airedale NHS Trust* vs *Bland* [1993] 1 All ER 821), the House of Lords upheld the declaration to withdraw nutrition and fluid (*Airedale NHS Trust* v. *Bland* [1993] 2 WLR 316) because, in the opinion of the medical team and his family, the treatment was futile as there was no hope that he would ever recover and therefore continuation of the treatment was not in his best interests.

Withdrawing nutrition support

In ethical terms, there is no distinction between withholding or withdrawing treatment (House of Lords, 1993). As nutrition support is classed as medical treatment it can be legally withdrawn if considered futile, but in practice it is often more difficult to stop feeding once started than for it not to have been provided at all. For this reason, there is sometimes a reluctance on the part of healthcare professionals to commence nutrition support for fear it will be difficult to stop. Where patients make that decision themselves, it should be respected, whatever the expected outcome.

Withdrawal or withholding nutrition support may be considered in cases where the patient has no prospect of recovery and continuation of the treatment will prolong the length of life but fail to improve the quality of that life to a standard acceptable to the patient. The BMA (2007) guidance states that:

> If treatment, including nutrition support and/or hydration, fails or ceases to give a net benefit to the patient, or if the patient has refused it – either contemporaneously or in advance – that goal cannot be realised and the justification for providing the treatment is removed.

In some cases, it may be appropriate to agree with the patient beforehand a point at which treatment will be stopped. Another option is to consider a trial over a specified period with the agreement that a review will be undertaken at the end of the trial or earlier if the patient's condition changes and that nutrition support will be stopped or adjusted, as appropriate.

The benefit of using these approaches, and including relatives and carers in discussions, is that the patient has the opportunity to discuss their concerns and gain a greater understanding of nutrition support and the implications for them, hopefully reducing misunderstandings at a later stage.

Any decision to actively withdraw nutrition and hydration must be reached through careful and thoughtful discussion, in consultation with relatives and in close discussion with everybody involved in the care of the patient.

Conclusion

Making sound clinical decisions regarding the provision of nutrition support can be challenging. Where conflict arises, a full multidisciplinary discussion is essential to explore the many ethical and legal pitfalls, including the patient and family, if appropriate. There are strong arguments both for and against the administration of nutrition support. The wishes of the patient are the primary guide for determining the treatment offered. In the case of an informed patient with decision-making capacity, their choice of non-treatment must be respected whatever the outcome of that decision. Where the patient is unable to participate in treatment decisions or their wishes are unknown, advice from family and carers should be sought to inform the decision-making process in the absence of an advanced directive.

References

Angus, F., Burakoff, R. (2003) The percutaneous endoscopic gastrostomy tube: Medical and ethical issues in placement. *American Journal of Gastroenterology* **92** (2), 272–7.

British Medical Association (2002) *Withholding and Withdrawing Life Prolonging Medical Treatment: Guidance for decision making*, Blackwell Publishing, London.

British Medical Association (2007) End of Life: Withdrawing and withholding nutrition support and hydration, www.bma.org.uk/ap.nsf/Content/endo flifewithdrawing?OpenDocument&Highlight=2,withdrawing,nutrition, accessed 23 January 2008.

Department of Health (2001a) *Good Practice in Consent Implementation Guide: consent to examination or treatment*, DH, London.

Department of Health (2001b) *Seeking Consent: Working with older people*, DH, London.

Department of Health (2005a) *Mental Capacity Act: Summary*, Department of Constitutional affairs, DH, London.

Department of Health (2005b) *Mental Capacity Act: Code of Practice*, Department of Constitutional Affairs, DH, London.

Dimond, B. (2005) *Legal Aspects of Nursing*, Pearson Education, London.

Dimond, B. (2007) The Mental Capacity Act and decision making: Best interests. *British Journal of Nursing* **16** (19), 1208–10.

Finucane, T.E., Christmas, C., Travis, K. (1999) Tube feeding in patients with advanced dementia: A review of the evidence. *Journal of the American Medical Association* **282** (14), 1365–70.

Hoefler, J.M. (2000) Making decisions about tube feeding for severely demented patients at the end of life: Clinical, legal and ethical considerations. *Death Studies* **24** (3), 233–54.

Hoffer, J.L. (2006) Analysis and comment controversy tube feeding in advanced dementia: The metabolic perspective. *British Medical Journal* **333**, 1214–15.

House of Lords (1993) *Report of the Select Committee on Medical Ethics*, Her Majesty's Stationery Office, London.

Keown, J. (2003) Medical murder by omission? The law and ethics of withholding and withdrawing treatment and tube feeding. *Clinical Medicine* **3** (5), 460–63.

Lennard-Jones, J.E. (1998) *Ethical and Legal Aspects of Clinical Hydration and Nutritional Support: A report by the working party of the British Association for Parenteral and Enteral Nutrition*, BAPEN, Maidenhead.

Lennard-Jones, J.E. (1999) Giving or withholding fluids and nutrients: Ethical and legal aspects. *Journal of the Royal College of Physicians* **33** (1), 39–45.

Li, I. (2002) Feeding tubes in patients with advanced dementia. *American Physician* **65** (8), 1605–10.

Macfie, J. (2001) Ethics and nutritional support therapy: A clinician's view. *Clinical Nutrition* **20** (1), 87–99.

McNamara, E.P., Kennedy, N.P. (2001) Tube feeding patients with advanced dementia: an ethical dilemma. *Proceedings of the Nutrition Society* **60** (2), 179–85.

Morris, C.H., Hope, R.A., Fairburn, C.G. (1989) Eating habits in dementia: A descriptive study. *British Journal of Psychiatry* **154**, 801–6.

National Institute for Health and Clinical Excellence (2006) *Nutrition Support in Adults: Oral nutrition support, enteral tube feeding and parenteral nutrition, Clinical Guideline 32*, NICE, London.

Nursing and Midwifery Council (2004) *NMC Code of Professional Conduct: Standards for conduct, performance and ethics*, NMC, London.

Sanders, D.S., Carter, M.J., D'Silva, J. *et al.* (2000) Survival analysis in percutaneous endoscopic gastrostomy feeding: A worse outcome in patients with dementia. *American Journal of Gastroenterology* **95** (6), 1472–5.

Smith, S.A., Andrews, M. (2000) Artificial nutrition and hydration at the end of life. *Medical Surgical Nursing* **9** (5), 233–42.

Young-In, K. (2001) To feed or not to feed: Tube feeding in patients with advanced dementia. *Nutrition Reviews* **59** (3), 86–8.

Further reading

Tingle, J., Cribb, A. (2007) *Nursing Law and Ethics*, Blackwell Publishing, London.

Tsaloglidou, A., Rammos, K., Kirlklidis, K. *et al.* (2007) Nurses' ethical decision-making role in nutrition support. *British Journal of Nursing* **16** (16), 996–1001.

Watson, R., Green, S. (2005) Feeding and dementia: A systematic literature review. *Journal of Advanced Nursing* **54** (1), 6–93.

Chapter 9

The Role of a Hospital Nutrition Support Team

Carolyn Best, Helen Hitchings, Joanna Boult and Harriet Gordon

Introduction

The provision of adequate and appropriate nutrition is the responsibility of all health professionals involved in caring for the patient admitted to hospital. However, for those patients who require nutrition support, particularly parenteral nutrition (PN), additional specialised support and advice are required to manage their nutritional needs. This is due to the complex issues that commonly arise in the provision and monitoring of the patient with PN, for example changes in biochemical status, difficulties in obtaining vascular access and increased infection risks.

It is considered best practice (Silk, 1994; Sizer, 1996; National Institute for Health and Clinical Excellence, 2006) that the needs of the patient requiring PN are met by a specialist multidisciplinary team: the Nutrition Support Team (NST). The NST is invaluable in ensuring the provision of nutrition support that is cost-effective and appropriate. The team is also well positioned to assess the suitability of nutrition support for individual patients and to highlight ethical dilemmas by offering specialist assessment (Reynolds *et al.*, 1995). The use of this team approach has been shown to improve standards in the provision of nutritional support and has been adopted by the British Association for Enteral and Parenteral Nutrition (BAPEN) as the recommended method of providing nutrition support throughout the United Kingdom (Powell-Tuck *et al.*, 1978; Silk, 1994).

In 2006, BAPEN (2006a) noted that less than half of all hospitals in the United Kingdom had an NST and urged hospital Trusts to ensure that an NST and a Nutrition Steering Committee (NSC) were either in place or in development by the first anniversary of the publication of the *Nutrition Support in Adults* guidelines (National Institute for Health and Clinical Excellence, 2006), i.e. February 2007. It argued that this would be the first step to ensuring that the best coordinated nutritional care in hospital would be available and accessible for all patients.

A systematic review undertaken by Naylor *et al.* (2004) showed that patients who have their nutritional needs managed by the NST receive appropriate levels of nutrition and experience a lower level of mechanical complications, whilst a controlled study undertaken by Dalton *et al.* (1984) demonstrated how patients managed by the NST have a lower level of catheter-insertion problems, catheter-related sepsis and achieve a lower level of PN-related metabolic complications than patients managed by their own medical team.

Other studies have shown (Anderson *et al.*, 1996; Trujillo *et al.*, 1999) that once the NST takes over responsibility for prescribing PN and monitoring its usage there is often a corresponding reduction in the level of inappropriate use and wastage.

Most NSTs have a core membership of a doctor, pharmacist, dietitian and a specialist nurse, or a combination of these disciplines. A number of other healthcare professionals may form part of a larger NST or provide additional support to decisions made by the team, including:

- biochemists
- microbiologists
- infection-control clinical nurse specialists
- speech and language therapists
- psychologists.

The approach and level of involvement in direct patient care of the NST will vary from organisation to organisation. They may take an advisory role at a strategic level but not be directly involved in day-to-day patient care, be more involved in an educative role or take on the active responsibility of managing a caseload of patients and prescribing nutrition support. However, Dalton *et al.* (1984) highlight how an NST that controls and supervises the administration of PN is able to provide a higher standard of care than an NST which only advises on the care that should be given.

Whatever level of support and advice the NST provides, its main purpose is to ensure the safe and effective delivery of PN to patients. Therefore, the responsibilities of the NST may involve some or all of the following:

- insertion and care of central catheters (for the provision of PN)
- prescribing PN
- evaluation and review of a patient's nutritional requirements
- fluid management
- compounding PN under aseptic conditions
- evaluation of drug therapy and its impact on the provision of PN
- advice on the safe administration of PN
- advice on the management of adverse reactions to PN
- negotiating with manufacturers to purchase products and services
- advice on complex issues around enteral nutrition support
- education and training
- research
- audit
- management of the home PN patient in the community.
  (Murphy & Scott, 2000)

Roles within the team

To promote accountability within the NST, it is imperative to clearly define the roles and responsibilities of each healthcare professional at the outset. Clear roles and responsibilities ensure the NST works to provide an effective and efficient support service. Whilst it is important that the team be flexible and can cover for one another during periods of sickness or annual leave, clear role definition is vital if team members are to advance their own knowledge and skills, develop the practice of other healthcare professionals and avoid confrontation and discontent.

It is useful to take time out to discuss roles at an early stage. Whether this is undertaken as part of a team-building day or something closer to home, by taking a couple of hours away from clinical responsibilities, it has to be decided at a local level. Whichever approach is used, it is essential this work is undertaken to ensure the future success of the NST.

Individual roles within the core team

The clinician

The NST clinician may be a gastroenterologist, a gastrointestinal (GI) surgeon, an intensivist or a chemical pathologist with an interest in nutritional problems who should have received specific training in nutrition support (National Institute for Health and Clinical Excellence, 2006). They should be of consultant basis and act as director of the team (Silk, 1994).

In practice, it is often a gastroenterologist who takes on the role of the NST clinician. This may be due to the fact that many of the patients referred for PN have some disease affecting the gut and that gastroenterologists often work closely with GI surgeons, who are often the referring clinician for PN (Burnham & Barton, 2001).

One study (Stockdale *et al.*, 1998) questioned 483 members of the British Society of Gastroenterologists (BSG) to determine the demands upon gastroenterologists for nutrition support. The study showed that of those consultants who participated 79% supervised patients on enteral feeding, 64% supervised PN and 27% headed, or were members of, an NST. The Royal College of Physicians (RCP; 2008) indicates that two hours per week should be allowed for rounds, and that the provision of the service should take up to two sessions per week.

The role of the clinician within the NST may include some or all of the following responsibilities:

- overall responsibility for the nutritional care of patients referred to the NST
- liaison with other clinicians to ensure effective communication and collaboration in the provision of care between the patient's medical team and the NST (Burnham & Barton, 2001)
- evaluation of the patient's pathophysiology (Hamilton, 2000)
- define the most suitable route of administration of nutrition support (Silk, 1994)
- discuss the ethics of nutrition support for individual patients with clinical colleagues (Silk, 1994)
- plan course of PN therapy, evaluate likely outcomes and period of duration of the PN required
- insertion, or supervision for the insertion, of central catheters (although in some areas this is increasingly being undertaken by nutrition nurse specialists)
- insertion of percutaneous endoscopic gastrostomy (PEG) tubes
- in collaboration with other members of the NST, ensure standards for nutrition support are met.

In practice, the resolution of ethical dilemmas may often be the most challenging aspect of the clinician's role, requiring close collaboration with diverse agencies, particularly relatives and medico-legal support (see Chapter Eight *passim*).

The pharmacist

The pharmacist's input within the NST is essential to standardise prescribing practices and documentation. This has been shown to decrease the incidence of prescribing errors in PN from 93% to 11% (White, 2003).

The pharmacist provides technical information and usually has a dual role: having a clinical input into the prescribing and monitoring of PN on the wards and being responsible for the production of the PN in the pharmacy.

Clinical role

The pharmacist attends the NST ward rounds primarily to assist in the prescribing of PN. The prescription is usually formulated using input from the team and the prescription signed by a doctor. However, the NST pharmacist may take on the extended role of a non-medical prescriber (as could the nutrition nurse specialist). Prescribing PN as a non-medical prescriber, the pharmacist would be responsible for writing the prescription themselves through the use of a clinical management plan and in agreement with the medical prescriber within the team.

Depending on local policy, members of the NST may be able to order blood tests for the patients receiving PN. Using these blood results, the pharmacist can adjust the electrolyte content of the prescription, where appropriate.

The pharmacist would also be involved in reviewing the patient's drug therapy where it is relevant to the prescription of PN, for example:

- querying the use of pro-kinetics where the patient has been diagnosed with ileus
- highlighting the use of prescribed diuretics to ensure the NST is aware of the need to closely monitor the patient's fluid-balance and electrolyte levels
- monitoring the patient for drug interactions which could affect the administration and prescription of PN, e.g. the use of warfarin or insulin (administration of PN containing vitamin K could cause warfarin resistance; increasing the rate of

administration of PN could affect the patient's blood-sugar
levels)
- highlighting patient discomfort resulting from medication side
  effects, e.g. nausea and vomiting following the use of opiate
  analgesia.

It is the responsibility of the pharmacist to draw the NST's attention
to these issues and where appropriate to the patient's supervising
medical team.

There should be close liaison between the ward-based pharmacist
and the NST pharmacist where a patient is either referred for nutrition
support or where it is being stopped. This ensures that there is an
ongoing review of the patient's prescribed medications and adjust-
ments are made as appropriate, for example initiating route-of-admin-
istration changes, such as switching oral medication to intravenous
or vice versa.

Commencing PN is never an emergency (National Institute for
Health and Clinical Excellence, 2006). The decision to start should be
planned, wherever possible. However, there may be occasions where
a decision to start PN is made out-of-hours, for example over the
weekend. In these circumstances the on-call pharmacist may be the
first person to give advice. Where appropriate access or blood results
are not available or the patient cannot be monitored closely, the advice
may include not starting PN at the time requested but making a
number of recommendations instead, including:

- requesting appropriate blood tests
- checking that the referring team has thought about the provision
  of appropriate central access
- commencing IV vitamins.

The patient would then be reviewed by the NST as soon as
possible.

Preparation of parenteral nutrition

The addition of vitamins and electrolytes is always carried out in a
specialist aseptic unit in a pharmacy, never within a clinical unit or
ward. This is due to the complex nature of this IV fluid. A contaminated infusion of PN would be a high infection risk to the patient.
Therefore, the use of a strict aseptic technique is essential during its
preparation.

The pharmacist in the aseptic unit receives the prescription from
the NST and calculates the volumes of ingredients required for the

formulation. The prescription should specify whether the NST requires a standard bag or one that will need to be tailored to an individual patient. It is fairly common practice to use standard bags of PN to which electrolytes, trace elements and vitamins are added.

If tailored PN is required for a patient, the pharmacist would formulate a product from scratch based on the level of calories, fat and protein the nutrition support dietitian has calculated the patient requires. Electrolytes, vitamins and trace elements could then be added.

The provision of a plain standard bag with no extra additions of electrolytes, vitamins and trace elements is not adequate for the patients starting PN (White, 2003); the risk of precipitating re-feeding syndrome would be too high. Therefore, only in exceptional circumstances and only with input from the NST should unsupplemented PN be supplied.

The pharmacist ensures that all the additives made to a bag of PN are compatible. PN infusions are extremely susceptible to becoming unstable when excess solutions are added. There is also a significant risk that a precipitate can be formed in the PN infusion, which, if unchecked, could go unnoticed in the opaque, white emulsion. Precipitation of PN is known to occur when calcium and phosphate solutions are added in incorrect amounts or added in rapid succession (Trissel, 2005). Therefore, it is imperative that strict checks are undertaken by the pharmacist during the preparation process to ensure this doesn't happen.

The nutrition nurse specialist

The role of the nutrition nurse specialist (NNS) is probably the key to the success of the NST, which is why in larger hospitals more than one NNS may be attached to the NST. In 2006, the National Institute for Health and Clinical Excellence (NICE) recommended that all acute hospitals should have at least one specialist nutrition support nurse in post. The input of the NNS is essential to develop protocols and implement standards for all nursing staff involved in providing patients with nutrition support.

A nurse specialist is an expert in a particular speciality or client group with post-qualification education in specialist clinical practice, care and programme management, clinical practice development and leadership (United Kingdom Central Council for Nursing, Midwifery and Health Visiting, 2002).

Depending on the demands of the service, the role of the NNS may vary from organisation to organisation. The NNS may be employed by an acute Trust and have sole responsibility for PN, whilst others will play a greater role in enteral nutrition support in hospital and the transfer of care into the community. Most NNSs have some level of responsibility in both parenteral and enteral nutrition support.

The key responsibilities of the NNS will include:

- providing expert clinical care
- being involved in and leading audit/research programmes
- teaching
- being an agent of change
- acting as the patient's advocate.
  (Silk, 1994; Miller, 1995)

Providing expert clinical care

The NNS will be both directly and indirectly involved in patient care.

Direct patient care activities will include:

- the assessment, organisation and support of patients requiring nutrition support
- the insertion of enteral feeding tubes:
  ○ first assistant in PEG insertion
  ○ percutaneous placement of balloon replacement gastrostomy and low-profile devices
- the insertion of peripherally inserted central catheters (PICCs)
- the repair and unblocking of access devices used for nutrition support.

Indirect care activities may include:

- providing education for healthcare professionals, patients and their families
- setting clinical standards for nutrition support
- developing evidence-based policies and guidelines for nutrition support
- reviewing and auditing clinical practice
- liaising with other healthcare professionals to give nursing advice
- providing ongoing support to the patient, their families and carers, and staff.

Audit/research

Responsibilities of the NNS in relation to audit and research include:

- analysing research relevant to nutrition support and considering its application to clinical practice
- disseminating research findings pertinent to nurses working with patients receiving nutrition support
- where appropriate, testing and applying the findings of research produced by others in the local care setting
- translating research findings into protocols and teaching sessions to promote the implementation of evidence-based practice
- leading or participating in audits/research relating to nutrition
- collaborating with other healthcare professionals to participate in national and international research projects relating to nutrition in hospitals.

Agent of change

This aspect of the role works hand in hand with that of the research as it involves incorporating valid and reliable research into clinical practice, promoting new ideas and reviewing and evaluating current practice.

Teaching

A large part of the provision of education in nutrition support will fall to the NNS. They will be responsible for ensuring nursing practice is evidence-based. Education may be provided in conjunction with other members of the NST, particularly the dietitian. As a result, the NNS will be involved to a greater or lesser degree in providing education to some or all of the following groups:

- registered nurses
- healthcare assistants
- nurses returning to practice
- link nurses
- medical students
- pharmacists
- dietitians
- medical staff
- allied health professionals

- community nursing services
- patients and their families and carers.

Education may be provided on both a formal and informal basis, to an individual or a group, for example teaching essential-skills training to a group of newly qualified nurses or one-on-one support to the patient going home on nutrition support. Where education is to develop a practical skill, for example the insertion of a nasogastric tube, it is useful to give the 'student' the opportunity to handle the equipment and practise the procedure on a mannequin. This provides a safe environment in which to make mistakes and ask questions.

For education to be effective, it is important to recognise that teaching sessions will not be a one-off event. They will need to be repeated at regular intervals to ensure staff and the patient/carer feel confident in their skills and knowledge and maintain a level of competence.

A number of issues will influence the level of knowledge within the clinical area, including:

- a high turnover of staff within a ward, resulting in a dilution in expertise
- infrequent admissions of patients requiring nutrition support; if a skill is not used regularly, levels of knowledge and hence competence fall, potentially resulting in the provision of inappropriate care and increasing stress levels in nursing staff
- historical care. We've all heard it at some point or other: 'This is the way we do it here' or 'We've always done it this way'. A continued programme of education can help to challenge out-of-date practice and provide support for junior staff.

It is important that clinical staff know how to access formal and ad hoc education from the NNS to inform and support their practice.

Topic areas commonly covered by an NNS will include:

- care of the patient with enteral nutrition support (including care of nasogastric, nasojejunal, gastrostomy or gastrojejunostomy feeding tubes)
- care of the patient with PN (including care of the central catheter)
- actions required to minimise complications relating to enteral and PN support
- ensuring adherence to nutrition support policies and guidelines
- discussing ethical issues which may arise in deciding whether to start (or stop) nutrition support

- practical aspects of assisting patients to eat
- providing support and information for the patient and family on the nutrition support relevant to them prior to discharge and liaison with community services.

Information given during teaching sessions must be evidence-based and, where requested, references must be provided to support this evidence. To support the knowledge imparted, it is often useful, particularly when teaching the patient and family, to provide written information as a back-up.

Acting as the patient's advocate

The NNS will often be the member of the NST in closest contact with the patient and family, especially in the early stages of organising access and setting up support services at home.

As a nurse, the NNS will be expected to promote the interests of patients within their care (Nursing and Midwifery Council, 2004). To undertake this role, the NNS will need to have a clear insight into the patient's wishes, needs and rights to represent their views to the wider healthcare team. When discussing proposals for care, the NNS must have an understanding of the proposed treatment and its implications for the patient, know who to refer them to for additional support and be able to provide clear, unbiased information to the patient and relatives upon which they can base their decision-making.

The role of the nutrition support dietitian

The NST dietitian is uniquely placed to give guidance and recommendations regarding the complex nutritional requirements of the patient requiring nutrition support and has an important part to play in the successful operating of an NST.

A nutrition support dietitian should be appropriately trained and experienced in the fields of nutrition assessment and nutrition support (Silk, 1994).

As with other roles within the NST, the dietitian needs to work collaboratively with ward staff, clinicians, patients and relatives, and often works within the team in a coordinator role.

Specific responsibilities of the nutrition support dietitian include:

- assessing actual nutritional intake, nutritional status and potential nutritional requirements

- consulting with other members of the NST about individual patients' need for nutrition support
- discussing nutritional requirements with other members of the NST, and how best to achieve these for individual patients – be it enteral or PN, or a combination of both
- translating patient requirements into a regimen that can be followed by ward staff
- translating nutritional requirements into a safe and practicable feeding regimen for individual patients
- assessing the risk of re-feeding syndrome in individual patients, and raising the awareness of the risks of re-feeding syndrome within the wider hospital population
- monitoring blood results and response to nutrition, in collaboration with other NST members
- playing an active role on the NSC within the hospital
- promoting the concept of nutrition support through education and training programmes for medical, nursing and other staff groups within the hospital independently or in conjunction with other members of the NST
- playing an important role in the decisions regarding which enteral and parenteral feeds are used within the hospital. This includes liaising with suppliers, medical equipment department, NNS and pharmacist
- training other dietitians with regard to nutrition support, and acting as a departmental and hospital resource when there are queries about nutrition support or about the best course of nutrition action for a patient.

Getting started: developing the Nutrition Support Team

The need to develop an NST may arise in response to clinical governance issues, the need to reduce spending on PN or from healthcare professionals with a role in nutrition support working in isolation recognising the need for support.

To maximise the chances of success, those working to develop an NST should try to use local problems to demonstrate the need for the team (Nightingale *et al.*, 1996; Nightingale & Reeves, 1999) and to build a business case. To make a successful business case, the individual must have a good knowledge of the evidence base for the proposal being made (Howard, 2001a). A healthcare library is often a good resource and can help in literature searches to provide supporting evidence.

Key stakeholders and allies will need to be identified at an early stage to assist and support the development of the NST and to increase awareness of organisational and service-level changes that will affect the new team's practice (Howard 2001a).

Key people to involve in the process at this point would include:

- dietitians (e.g. chief dietitian, any nutrition support dietitian already in post)
- chief pharmacist responsible for PN
- clinicians (e.g. gastroenterologist, intensivist, general physicians and general surgeons)
- nurses (e.g. directors of nursing in both secondary and primary care, senior nurses).

Other links that may be useful include:

- clinical effectiveness and audit team
- medical librarian (see above)
- catering manager
- business manager
- laboratory staff
- BAPEN regional representatives.

The task of rationalising nutrition support practices to provide a coherent process that supports all healthcare professionals without causing upset and discontent is not going to be easy. Good communication, careful planning, sensitive implementation and robust monitoring are essential (Howard, 2001b).

To function effectively, the newly formed NST will need to clearly explain to all relevant health professionals and clinical areas:

- how and why to refer to the NST
- how the involvement of the NST will affect their workload
- what benefits referral to the NST will give them
- how effective communication channels will be developed and maintained.

Agreeing the referral process

It is important to develop a referral process that is simple to use and easy to remember.

The referral criteria should include:

- who is able to make a referral (e.g. ward nurses, dietitians, pharmacists, junior doctors)
- what information is needed (e.g. patient details, medical conditions, whether central access is already available or will need to be arranged)
- what investigations should have been made in preparation (e.g. full blood count (FBC), urea and electrolytes (U & Es), liver-function tests (LFTs), phosphate, magnesium and calcium levels, patient weight).

Developing skills within the Nutrition Support Team

The NST will be regularly involved in providing education for other healthcare professionals, but in order to be able to do this effectively and provide the most up-to-date information it is essential that they have the opportunity to develop their own skills and knowledge. As the founder organisation for nutrition support, BAPEN offers support and education at a local and national level. Each discipline within the core team has an affiliate group within BAPEN:

- BAPEN Medical (clinicians)
- BPNG: the British Pharmaceutical Nutrition Group (pharmacists)
- NNNG: the National Nurses Nutrition Group (nurses)
- PENG: the Parenteral and Enteral Nutrition Group of the British Dietetic Association (dietitians).

Members of the NST should use these resources to develop their own knowledge both as a group and as individuals.

Maintaining momentum

Once the initial excitement of developing the team is over, it may be challenging to keep focused, particularly if members of the team do not have a clearly defined purpose or cannot be regularly involved in the team's work. Organisational change and staff leaving are the most common reasons for a team to flounder (Howard, 2001a). Therefore, the NST should be committed to its own development as much as it is to the care of the patients referred to it (Howard, 2001b). Meeting regularly, and with an agreed agenda, is invaluable to this process. It is important to develop an action plan not only for the NST's day-to-day activity but also for the education of team members and the development of practice on a wider level throughout the team's area of responsibility. It is important for the newly developed NST to recognise this will be an ongoing process. Individuals within the NST may become despondent when initiatives do not move as quickly as they would like or there is a resistance to a recommended change in practice. The key to being successful in improving nutrition practices is to be clinically involved in those with complex nutritional needs and to be visible to those whose practice we are trying to influence.

A lack of motivation within the NST can result in reduced standards of patient care, which will have a demoralising effect on both the patient and the medical and nursing teams caring for them (Hamilton, 2000).

In time, where the workload for one NST may become too great, it may be necessary to explore the development of further teams with areas of specific responsibility, for example intensive-care units and paediatrics, but development should only be taken one step at a time and in achievable chunks.

Agreeing standards for practice

As a starting point, it would be advisable for the NST to explore what policies, guidelines or care plans relating to nutrition are already in place, how they were developed and circulated, who was/is responsible for updating them and how effective they are at influencing nutrition practice. It is advisable to collaborate with the individual concerned to introduce the remit of the newly developed NST and decide whether members of the NST take over the responsibility for the development of policies and standards or just participate in the process in an advisory capacity.

Suggested areas to explore may include the use of:

- screening tools
- food handling/hygiene policies
- guidelines on assisting patients to eat
- the provision of enteral nutrition, including tube care
- the provision of PN and insertion/care of central and peripheral catheters

- nutrition monitoring (e.g. food and fluid charts)
- infection-control policies.

There will be extensive knowledge and skills within the NST itself. Some members of the team may have previously held responsibilities for the development of nutrition-related policies and guidelines but have worked on them in isolation. With input from all members of the NST, newly developed policies and guidelines should reflect the multidisciplinary approach required to tackle nutrition issues and be more relevant to practice situations and promote evidence-based practice (Schneider, 2006).

To increase the chances of your guidelines being used in clinical areas, they should be clear, concise and accessible. Large tomes are likely to sit getting dusty upon a shelf!

Once the NST has a clear idea of the necessary work involved for the development of policies and guidelines, the team will need to explore other areas of practice, including:

- how the provision of enteral feeding is organised in the hospital. This should include information on:
  - the number and types of feed solutions used
  - who is responsible for the delivery and care of equipment (e.g. enteral feeding pumps)
  - feeding tubes: how are they financed, who holds responsibility for ordering them and where they are stored
  - how often the service is reviewed
- how the provision of PN is organised. This should include information on:
  - solutions (as above)
  - intravenous feeding lines: what types of line are used, who is responsible for insertion
  - aseptic services: how are they provided (i.e. in-house or whether PN is ordered through another hospital or PN company)
  - volumetric pumps (as above)
  - how often the service is reviewed
- who holds the budget in both the hospital and the community
  - for enteral tube feeding
  - for parenteral solutions
  - for delivery systems
  - for ancillaries
  - for feeding lines/tubes
  - for pumps

- what procedures are in place for discharging patients into the community with nutrition support
- who is trained to pass fine-bore nasogastric tubes in the hospital and in the community and what procedures are in place to guide them
- who holds the responsibility for arranging placement and placing PEGs and replacement feeding tubes in the hospital and in the community and what procedures are in place to guide them
- who inserts parenteral feeding lines
- which meetings are important to attend
- whether there have been any problems identified in the management and provision of nutrition support
- what is available in terms of clerical support, access to computer facilities and educational support (to attend meetings either as a team or individually).
(British Association for Parenteral and Enteral Nutrition, 2006b)

Proving the worth of the Nutrition Support Team

Clinical audit

The survival of the NST rests on its ability to demonstrate improved patient outcomes, reduced healthcare costs and complication rates in relation to nutrition support. Therefore, auditing practice is an important issue that should be integral to the work of the team. It is advisable to start the process by auditing those areas of practice the team is aiming to improve. The NST is in an ideal position to audit local practice against national guidelines, to identify gaps in service provision and to implement essential guidelines and procedures to improve practice.

Although the inception of an NST may actually increase rather than decrease the use of PN, as usage becomes more appropriate it may be possible to identify cost savings. By comparing the use of PN before the development of the NST with its projected use (by the NST), savings may be identified in a number of areas.

Examples of audit topics that could be easily undertaken by the NST include:

- the number of referrals received for PN/PEG insertion
- the numbers of patients who receive PN/PEG insertion
- the numbers of patients who refuse PN/PEG insertion
- when PN/PEG is refused or not recommended, which alternative routes of feeding are there

- waiting times for central catheter or enteral feeding tube insertion
- number of bags of PN used per patient; Kennedy and Nightingale (2005) show how cost savings were made by an NST in the number of PN episodes that were avoided
- the number of and reasons why bags of PN are wasted
- average length of feeding
- catheter-related sepsis: this has been found to lessen with the introduction of a nutrition nurse (Keohane *et al.*, 1983; Kennedy & Nightingale, 2005)
- metabolic complications
- length of time PN is used before enteral nutrition is introduced
- number of blood requests made
- pharmacist time in the preparation unit
- medication costs.

Financing the Nutrition Support Team

The financing of the NST will depend on how it was set up. It may be funded as a separate entity or part funded within individual job descriptions. If team members are funded in terms of hours, it is vital to ensure that those hours are ring-fenced and other responsibilities do not impede.

Team budget

At a basic level, a budget will be required to fund the equipment needed to provide nutrition support, for example central lines and replacement ends for feeding tubes. However, even without access to a large budget, the NST can advise on cost-effectiveness during the purchase of equipment for nutrition support and participate in contract negotiations to evaluate enteral or parenteral feeding options.

Team fund

The setting-up of a team fund can be useful for providing finance for educational purposes. In the current healthcare climate, it is not always easy to obtain funding for continuing education from employing organisations. Participation in outside educational programmes, writing articles for publication and involvement in research projects include some of the ways the NST can generate income for education.

Team meetings and annual reviews

Regular team meetings are essential to collate ongoing audits, review goals and standards previously set, and to identify improvements in services or problems (both financial and clinical) that may be developing. They also serve to nudge team members into remembering which projects they should be leading as the day-to-day work has a habit of taking over! Writing an annual report allows the team time to reflect on and recognise its successes as well as providing a base upon which to plan initiatives for the following year.

The annual report should summarise activity over the previous year, for example:

- PEGs: number of referrals, placements and problems encountered
- PN: number of referrals, number actually receiving PN, number of bags wasted etc.

It should describe the main goals for that year and whether or not they have been achieved. This is an ideal time to summarise costs for the year, savings and projected needs for the next year. The data held year on year are helpful in reminding management that the NST is actually self-funding and not an area where cutting services will provide hospital savings.

Publicising success

To ensure the survival and continued development of the NST, it is essential to publicise the work of the team, particularly when it can enhance the image of the organisation. At a local level, publicity may be in the form of newsletters, grand rounds or annual reports highlighting, for example, a reduction in complications for PN or cost savings. At a national level, it may mean becoming involved in developing a poster or presenting at a national conference or writing articles for inclusion in a journal. Not publicising the successes of the team may over a period of time lead to a poor understanding of its purpose, leading to a lessening of the support and interest of strategic bodies and decision-makers.

The role of the Nutrition Steering Committee

NICE (2006) states that each Trust should have an NSC as part of the clinical governance framework, chaired by Trust management, with representation from catering, pharmacy, dietetics and nursing as well as the NST. The remit of the NSC is to look at nutrition on a wider level than the NST and to create the opportunity for communication between all those involved in the nutritional care of patients. Silk (1994) recommends that the NSC should meet at least twice a year.

The first priority of the NSC is to provide a multidisciplinary approach which ensures the provision of food to the patient that is of a high standard, is palatable, in the correct format (for example soft or purée), and is served in an appropriate and timely manner (Silk, 1994). There must be close working with the NST, as the NSC's second priority involves ensuring that patients who need nutrition support receive it in an appropriate and timely manner.

In addition to these, the NSC should be responsible for:

- submitting business plans for catering and nutrition support to the chief executive
- negotiating catering and NST budgets
- liaising with regional services to ensure that hospital purchasing authorities include contract specifications for hospital catering and nutrition support
- ensuring standards for hospital catering and nutrition support are developed and adhered to
- setting standards for nutrition assessment
- establishing appropriate systems for referral
- implementing an agreed process for the auditing of catering and nutrition support services (Silk, 1994).

Conclusion

There are a number of benefits to the patient and the employing organisation of developing an NST. A well-managed and proactive multidisciplinary NST will raise awareness of the importance of nutrition support, enhance patient management and improve standards of nutritional care whilst often making considerable financial savings.

References

Anderson, C., Heimburger, D., Morgan, D.C. (1996) Metabolic complication of total parenteral nutrition: effects of a nutrition support service. *Journal of Parenteral and Enteral Nutrition* **20**, 106–210.

British Association for Enteral and Parenteral Nutrition (2006a) Press release: Hospitals missing target on required Nutrition Support Teams, 26th October 2006, www.bapen.org.uk/res_press_rel21.html, accessed 5 January 2008.

British Association for Enteral and Parenteral Nutrition (2006b) Education Training: For joining an established nutrition support team or introducing a nutritional support service, www.bapen.org.uk/res_educ_train_nut_team.html, accessed 8 January 2008.

Burnham, R., Barton, S. (2001) The Role of the Nutrition Support Team, in *Artificial Nutrition Support in Clinical Practice*, 2nd edn (eds J. Payne-James, G. Grimble, D.B.A Silk), Cambridge University Press, Cambridge.

Dalton, M.J., Schepers, G., Gee, J.P. *et al.* (1984) Consultative total parenteral nutrition teams: The effect on the incidence of total parenteral nutrition-related complications. *Journal of Parenteral and Enteral Nutrition* **8** (2), 146–52.

Hamilton, H. (2000) *Total Parenteral Nutrition: A Practical Guide for Nurses*, Churchill Livingstone, London.

Howard, P. (2001a) Keynote Lecture 2: Practical nutritional support: Working together to make it happen. *Proceedings of the Nutrition Society* **60**, 415–18.

Howard, P. (2001b) Organisational aspects of starting and running an effective nutritional support service. *Clinical Nutrition* **20** (4), 367–74.

Kennedy, J.F., Nightingale, J.M.D. (2005) Cost savings of an adult nutrition support team. *Nutrition* **21** (11/12), 1127–33.

Keohane, P.P., Jones, B.J.M., Attrill, H. *et al.* (1983) Effect of catheter tunnelling and a nutrition nurse on catheter sepsis during parenteral nutrition: A controlled trial. *Lancet* **2**, 1388–90.

Miller, L. (1995) The clinical nurse specialist: a way forward? *Journal of Advanced Nursing* **22**, 494–501.

Murphy, A., Scott, A. (2000) Artificial nutritional support: What are the options? *Hospital Pharmacist* **7** (6), 146–54.

National Institute for Health and Clinical Excellence (2006) *Nutrition Support in Adults: Oral nutrition support, enteral tube feeding and parenteral nutrition, Clinical Guideline 32*, NICE, London.

Naylor, C.J., Griffiths, R.D., Fernandez, R.S. (2004) Does a multidisciplinary Total Parenteral Team improve patient outcomes? A systematic review. *Journal of Parenteral and Enteral Nutrition* **28** (4) , 251–8.

Nightingale, J., Reeves, J. (1999) Knowledge about the assessment and management of undernutrition: A pilot questionnaire in a UK teaching hospital. *Clinical Nutrition* **18** (1), 23–7.

Nightingale, J.M.D., Walsh, N., Bullock, M.E., Wicks, A.C. (1996) Three simple methods of detecting malnutrition on medical wards. *Journal of the Royal Society of Medicine* **89** (3), 144–8.

Nursing and Midwifery Council (2004) *The NMC Code of Professional Conduct: Standards for conduct, performance and ethics*, NMC, London.

Powell-Tuck, J., Neilsen, T., Farwell, J.A., Lennard-Jones, J.E. (1978) Team approach to long term intravenous feeding in patients with gastrointestinal disorders. *Lancet* **2**, 825.

Reynolds, N., McWhirter, J.P., Pennington, C.R. (1995) Nutrition support teams: An integral part of developing a gastroenterology service. *Gut* **37** (6), 740–2.

Royal College of Physicians (2008) *Consultant Physicians Working for Patients: Gastroenterology*, 4th edn, RCP, London.

Schneider, P.J. (2006) Nutrition Support Teams: An evidence based practice. *Nutrition in Clinical Practice* **21** (1), 62–7.

Silk, D.B.A. (1994) *Organisation of Nutritional Support in Hospitals: Nutrition steering committee and nutrition support teams: Needs, structure and roles. A report by a working party of the British Association for Parenteral and Enteral Nutrition*, BAPEN, Maidenhead.

Sizer, T. (1996) *Standards and Guidelines for Nutritional Support of Patients in Hospitals. A report by a working party of the British Association for Parenteral and Enteral Nutrition*, BAPEN, Maidenhead.

Stockdale, A.C., Williams, B., Pennington, C.R. (1998) The role of the gastroenterologist in the provision of artificial nutrition support. *Alimentary Pharmacology & Therapeutics* **12** (4), 367–72.

Trissel, L.A. (2005) *Handbook on Injectable Drugs*, 13th edn, American Society of Health-System Pharmacists, Bethesda, MD.

Trujillo, E.B., Young, L.S., Chertow, G.M. *et al.* (1999) Metabolic and monetary costs of avoidable parenteral nutrition use. *Journal of Parenteral and Enteral Nutrition* **23** (2), 109–13.

United Kingdom Central Council for Nursing, Midwifery and Health Visiting (2002) *Report of the Higher Level of Practice Pilot and Project*, UKCC, London.

White, R. (2003) The role of the pharmacist in clinical nutrition. *Complete Nutrition* **3** (5), 21–3.

Chapter 10

Transfer of Care from Hospital to Community

Carolyn Best and Helen Hitchings

Introduction

This chapter will examine some of the issues that arise when patients who require home enteral feeding are discharged from hospital into their own homes or into a care home. It is recognised that some patients will attend the hospital only for the insertion of a feeding tube and be discharged home the same day. Although direct reference to these patients is not made, the issues and problems that may arise are similar to those of patients discharged from hospital.

Planning discharge

There are a number of benefits to providing home enteral feeding, including improved patient well-being and cost savings (Elia *et al.*, 1994). However, problems will arise if care is not taken to arrange appropriate aftercare and training. Planning for discharge should start as soon as possible following the decision that long-term artificial enteral feeding is required. This is essential to facilitate the organisation and care necessary for patients requiring enteral feeding in the community. Most patients will receive their feed through a gastrostomy, but jejunostomy and nasogastric tubes may be used for some patients where post-pyloric feeding is required or insertion of a gastrostomy is not an option. It is important that, where possible, the patient is established on a feeding regimen that meets their nutritional requirements prior to discharge. Unfortunately, with the ever-present pressure on hospital beds patients may be discharged before a feeding regimen is established. Effective liaison with community health and social care teams is essential to ensure such patients, and their carers or care home staff, receive adequate support and ongoing monitoring upon discharge (Stroud *et al.*, 2003).

Home enteral nutrition allows the patient to return to a familiar environment where support can be provided by family, friends or carers. It is important, however, that the burdens of home enteral feeding are made clear to all parties before being allowed home. The patient will have probably been made aware of the fact that a feeding tube will allow them to receive fluid and nutrition appropriate to their needs, but they are not always informed that initially they may be attached to a pump for at least 12–16 hours a day until the risk of re-feeding syndrome has passed and their feeding regimen is established and is meeting their nutritional requirements. Although this may paint a fairly bleak picture in the early stages of feeding, it is important to state that this may not always be the case. With careful planning, it is possible for patients to return to work or education.

Feed can be continuously delivered via a mobile pump, which can be carried in a specially designed rucksack or be administered via a syringe (bolus) at agreed time slots convenient to the individual. For such patients, consideration may need to be given to the type of feeding tube present. A button gastrostomy or low-profile device would be a more discreet option than a balloon gastrostomy, percutaneous endoscopic gastrostomy (PEG) tube or nasogastric tube.

All patients on home enteral feeding should be registered on the British Artificial Nutrition Survey (BANS). The BANS monitors the numbers of patients receiving artificial nutrition support in the community throughout the United Kingdom. Consent should be obtained from the patient to register them with BANS before discharge.

BANS produces regular reports from the data submitted, which can show trends, for example the increasing number of enterally fed patients living in the community.

Education

Although education will be provided whilst the patient is in hospital, it is often an extremely steep learning curve for the patient or carer once in their own home. They do not have the immediate support of ward staff to rely upon and may become extremely anxious at having to manage alone. It is important to ensure that the patient and their family are aware of the support that is available to them in the community and are provided with contact names and numbers for the relevant services.

Patients and/or their carers must be trained so that they feel confident and competent in administering feed and caring for the feeding tube in the simplest, safest and most effective way for them. Training should start as early as possible so that potential problems can be identified and mistakes made whilst support is available. Some patients may attend day centres, special schools or respite facilities. Not all staff in such facilities are trained or willing to administer feed or medication, but it is often beneficial to provide some basic education to raise the awareness of staff on how the feeding tube is used and what actions or omissions will cause a problem for the patient.

Training required

Where possible, it is advisable to train more than one person on how to care for the feed and tube to ensure that if problems arise or the patient becomes unable to care for the feed themselves there is another person who can take over responsibility for feeding.

If the patient is in hospital, training often falls to the nurse on the ward. Relevant hospital policies/guidelines should be referred to before advising the patient to ensure the most appropriate and relevant information is given. Suggested issues to cover can be seen in Box 10.1.

Box 10.1   Topics to be covered in training sessions

---

1. The reason why enteral tube feeding is required
2. The type of feeding tube the patient has in situ and the care it requires
3. How to administer the feed (is bolus or continuous/pump feeding to be used?)
4. Pump training (if required)
5. How much feed to give and how often
6. How to administer medications
7. Whether or not oral intake is permitted
8. How to flush the feeding tube
9. Why regular flushing is necessary
10. How and where feed should be stored
11. How to obtain enteral feed and disposable items
12. How often giving sets and syringes should be replaced
13. Troubleshooting measures, e.g.:
    - What action to take if a pump malfunctions
    - How to unblock a feeding tube
14. Who is responsible for providing continuing support and review

Equipment required for discharge

For home enteral feeding to be successful, prior to being discharged the patient will need to be supplied with an adequate amount of feed and equipment until their prescription and delivery can be organised in the community. This may take up to seven days to organise. Therefore, the patient should be discharged from hospital with:

- at least seven days of suitable feed
- syringes of the appropriate size (a 50 ml syringe is normally used for flushing, whilst a smaller syringe may be required for the administration of medication; purple enteral syringes should be used for the administration of all medication via an enteral feeding tube)
- a written feed regimen
- literature about the care of the tube and pump and the setting-up of a feed
- a feeding pump and stand (if required)
- contact details for:
  o   feed enquiries
  o   problems with the feeding tube
  o   problems with the pump.

Enteral feeds in the community are available on prescription, but the feeding equipment, or 'plastics', such as syringes, is generally financed by the community budget, either the district nursing budget or nursing home if the patient is a resident. To avoid difficulties in obtaining supplies post discharge, confirmation of who pays for the 'plastics' must be established before a patient is discharged.

Most UK feeding companies can provide training for patients, carers and care staff on their own equipment, arrange delivery of feed and feeding equipment to the patient's home, or care home, and provide servicing of pumps.

The review process

Healthcare professionals often assume that patients or carers of long-term home enterally fed patients are competent in administering feeds. However, skills in administering feeds, medication or fluid via an enteral tube should be reviewed in the home on a regular basis to ensure correct techniques are maintained and problems identified at an early stage to avoid tube blockage or damage to the tube. The patient's clinical condition may change, making it either more or less likely that they are able to cope with the feed themselves.

During the first weeks of managing at home, the level of support and review may be intense as the patient settles on a feeding regimen and becomes familiar with the care required to provide their enteral feed. As they become more familiar with the process and gain in confidence and competence, the professional input required to support them will gradually lessen.

Regular monitoring can result in significant benefits for the patient, carers and healthcare professionals, including:

- increased confidence and empowerment
- reduced incidence of complications
- nutritional requirements more likely to be met
- reduced incidence of severe electrolyte and metabolic abnormalities
- cost savings (Gales & Gales, 1994).

Initial review

Initial reviews should include discussion around some or all of the following:

1. Has there been clear communication from secondary to primary care services?
2. Are all the appropriate healthcare professionals involved?
3. What support are they providing?
4. Is all the necessary equipment available?
5. Is the patient able to tolerate the level of nutrition support being provided/recommended?
6. Does it fit in with their lifestyle?
7. Does the patient and/or carer feel able to cope with the task?
8. Does the feeding regimen need to be manipulated in view of medications/change in clinical condition/tolerance of feed?

Once nutrition support is established, monitoring should be undertaken as appropriate to the individual patient. Some factors may indicate the need for increasing the frequency of monitoring (Box 10.2).

Box 10.2   Clinical indications for increasing the frequency of monitoring

---

1. Changes in clinical condition/treatment
2. Changes in oral intake
3. A deterioration or improvement in swallow
4. Changes in nutritional status
5. The development of pressure ulcers
6. Localised or systemic infections
7. Biochemical abnormalities
8. Malabsorption
9. Poor feed tolerance: may result in receiving suboptimal levels of feed
10. Feeding regimens which do not provide recommended daily allowances for vitamins or minerals
11. Patients receiving additional vitamins or electrolytes
12. Recent discharge from hospital
13. Tube complications

Ongoing review

Ongoing patient review should include assessing:

- changes in the patient's clinical condition
- changes in prescribed or over-the-counter medication, including:
  - the method of administration
  - dose
  - timing in relation to feeding
  - whether a break in feeding is necessary
- whether the patient and/or carer is still competent to:
  - administer feed, flushes or medication appropriately
  - care for the feeding tube
- the feeding tube and stoma site (Table 10.1)
- whether referral to other healthcare professionals is required, e.g. speech and language therapist, occupational therapist.

When requesting an enteral feed prescription from a GP, it is recommended that the following are monitored, as appropriate:

- **Weight:** monthly where possible. Where weighing the patient is not an option, other measures may prove useful, such as mid-upper-arm circumference (MUAC), tricep-skinfold thickness

Table 10.1 Review of feeding tube and stoma site

The feeding tube

Look at:

- The condition of the tube:
  - Does it show signs of flattening, bubbling or discolouration?
  - How long has the tube been in place?
  - When is it due to be replaced?
  - Can it be replaced at home or is referral to hospital required?
- Is the tube correctly positioned?
  - Check the position of the bumper or flange
  - Check for tube migration
- Does the position of the tip of the tube need to be checked regularly (e.g. a nasogastric tube)?
- If the patient has a PEG, can the tube be advanced into the abdomen and rotated? (Do not rotate without advancing the tube. Buried bumper can still occur.)
- Do PEG attachments need to be replaced?

The stoma site

Look at:

- The condition of the stoma:
  - Does it look healthy?
  - Are there signs of inflammation, infection or exudate?
  - Does the patient complain of discomfort?
- If exudate is present is it due to:
  - infection?
  - gastric leakage?
  - poor positioning of the tube?
- Is a dressing used?
  - Is it an appropriate use of a dressing?
  - Is it changed at appropriate intervals?

NB: If the site is clean and dry, no dressing is required around gastrostomy tube.

(TSF), mid-arm-muscle circumference (MAMC) or hand-grip dynomometry.

- **Blood profile:** urea and electrolytes (U & Es), liver-function tests (LFTs), renal function and haemoglobin (Hb).

If a patient is discharged home prior to full feeding being established, more regular blood monitoring for the avoidance of re-feeding syndrome may be required. This is also necessary to ensure that the dietitian is able to increase nutritional intake in line with re-feeding guidelines (National Institute for Health and Clinical Excellence, 2006). In such cases, magnesium, phosphate and calcium would also need to be monitored, and thiamine prescribed.

If any abnormal results are received, for example a low serum sodium, a urinary sodium concentration check would be recommended prior to commencing any replacement therapy.

There are no prospective randomised controlled trials to determine which parameters should be measured and how often during artificial nutrition support (Fettes, 2004). Until the National Institute for Health and Clinical Excellence's (NICE; 2006) guidelines on nutrition support in adults, there were no national recommendations for what should be monitored and how often. NICE now has a protocol for laboratory monitoring in nutrition support. This includes the rationale for including the test, interpretation of results and the frequency of monitoring.

It is advisable to monitor daily U & Es, phosphate, calcium and magnesium three times a week, during the initial stages of feeding when regular alterations to feeding regimens are commonplace, owing to the risk of re-feeding syndrome and patient tolerance. Once the patient's blood levels are stable, the frequency of these tests can be reduced.

Potential problems

A number of problems may occur, especially during the first couple of weeks following discharge whilst the patient and their family are learning to care for the feeding tube and feeding regimen. Appropriate support is vital during this period, but once the patient is established and becomes confident in managing their nutritional needs the support required will lessen.

Poor communication

For the safe transfer of the patient, there must be a clear channel of communication between healthcare professionals in secondary and primary care services.

Staff who may be involved in the patient's care once they are discharged from hospital include:

- community dietitians
- speech and language therapists
- nutrition nurse specialists
- district nurses
- GPs
- feed company nurses/reps
- budget holder for plastics.

Before the patient is discharged, it is essential that all key community healthcare professionals are contacted by telephone and in writing. This communication should begin as early as possible, as community staff may request/require training on the care of feeding tubes or enteral feeding pumps.

Lack of support

Lack of support may occur if there has not been effective communication between secondary and primary care services before discharging the patient. If the patient feels unsupported, they are likely to feel less confident in managing their enteral feeding alone, leading to increased contacts with the GP, district nurses and hospital services.

Pressure on hospital beds often leads to early discharge into the community of enterally fed patients, and so it is important that patients are reviewed regularly during the initial period to ensure optimum nutrition support is received.

Patient support groups such as PINNT (Patients on Intravenous and Nasogastric Therapy) and LITRE (looking into requirements for equipment) may be useful for some patients.

Storage space for supplies

This may be an issue for patients and their carers as feed is often delivered on a monthly basis. This means that a large number of boxes of feed will be delivered at one time. Add to this syringes, giving sets and other consumables and it is easy to see why storage becomes an issue. A homecare company can deliver food directly to the patient's home or care home. Without this service, feed will need to be collected from, or delivered by, a pharmacy.

Some patients may store their feed in a garage. Care needs to be taken to ensure the feed is brought into the house to warm in the colder months because the administration of feed stored at a cold temperature may cause abdominal discomfort.

Inability to obtain all feed supplies

It is usually advisable to ensure that patients have a small buffer stock of feed and equipment that will last for three to four days. This ensures that if for any reason a delivery cannot be made, or a pharmacy has difficulty obtaining a certain feed, the patient is still able to continue feeding.

It requires good prescription management to ensure patients request repeat prescriptions in a timely fashion. This can also be one benefit of using a home feed delivery system as often the company will assume responsibility for communicating with a patient, and completing a stock check. They will also alert the dietitian if a stock check reveals a discrepancy between the expected and actual usage of feeds.

Breakdown of equipment

Using a homecare company

When pumps are supplied by a homecare company, it is usually a requirement that they be checked on an annual basis to ensure they remain safe to use. This should minimise the risk of a pump breaking down. However, in the event of a pump malfunctioning, a substitute is usually provided within 24 to 48 hours. Some homecare companies provide their own nurse to help with training and provide support to patients using their equipment.

Without the support of a homecare company

Some Primary Care Trusts purchase their own pumps for use by their patients. They will have their own guidelines for replacing damaged or malfunctioning pumps and for providing training on how to use the pump.

However, if this system is used, it is advisable to have a framework in place so that should a problem with a pump arise outside of normal office hours there is a means to resolve the issue and continue enteral feeding.

If a patient is unable to obtain a replacement pump out of hours, they need to be able to administer feed either via gravity or bolus, to ensure they remain hydrated when enteral feeding is their only means of hydration. Patients or their carers may therefore require information or education regarding this.

Sleep disturbance

This may be an issue for those patients who are fed overnight and involves the noise of the pump delivering the feed and possible occlusion or discomfort caused by lying on the feeding tube. This in turn may cause the pump to alarm. The patient may also feel the need to urinate more frequently and so may need to disconnect the feed to get to the bathroom. This should be explained to the patient prior to commencing overnight feeding, as trying to get across a room without disconnecting the feed could be potentially hazardous for the patient in a semi-awake state.

Blocked feeding tubes

The risk of tube blockage can be minimised by providing education for the patient and carers prior to discharge and by ensuring there is ongoing review once home enteral feeding is firmly established. It is often helpful to provide written information which can be referred to should a problem arise.

Conclusion

The provision of enteral tube feeding at home increases year on year, with patients being discharged from hospital to manage their nutrition in their own homes or in care homes before regimens have been established.

To ensure the discharge process goes smoothly, i.e. that adequate training is provided and appropriate services are set up, it is essential that discharge planning is commenced as early as possible and that there is clear communication between all acute and community services. A poor or hastily arranged discharge may result in the patient being admitted back to hospital for something that, with a little more time or explanation, could have been managed at home.

References

Elia, M., Cottee, S., Holden, C. *et al.* (1994) *Enteral and Parenteral Nutrition in the Community: A report by a working party of the British Association for Parenteral and Enteral Nutrition*, BAPEN, Maidenhead.

Fettes, S. (2004) Monitoring, in *A Pocket Guide to Clinical Nutrition 2004*, (eds. V. Todovoric, A. Micklewright), British Dietetic Association, London.

Gales B.J., Gales M.J. (1994) Nutrition Support Teams: A review of comparative trials. *The Annals of Pharmacotherapy* **28**, 227–35.

National Institute for Health and Clinical Excellence (2006) *Nutrition Support in Adults: Oral nutrition support, enteral tube feeding and parenteral nutrition, Clinical Guideline 32*, NICE, London.

Stroud, M., Duncan, H., Nightingale, J. (2003) Guidelines for enteral feeding in adult hospital patients. *Gut* **52** (Supplement VII), vii1–vii12.

Further reading

Clinical Resource Efficiency Support Team (2004) *Guidelines for the management of enteral tube feeding in adults*, CREST, Belfast.

Mensforth A., Spalding D. (1998) Discharge planning for home enteral tube feeding. *Clinical Nutrition Update* **3** (2), 8–10.

Support group details

BANS: British Artificial Nutrition Survey, Streets Heaver Healthcare Computing, 4 Low Moor Road, Lincoln LN6 3BR; access reports via BAPEN website (www.bapen.org).

LITRE: access via BAPEN website www.bapen.org.uk ('About us/members' organisations').

PINNT: Patients on Intravenous and Nasogastric Nutrition Therapy, PO Box 3126, Christchurch, Dorset BH23 2XS, United Kingdom; website: www. pinnt.com.

Chapter 11

Case Studies

Harriet Gordon, Carolyn Best, Helen Hitchings and Joanna Boult

Introduction

Within this chapter, we will present a selection of cases which highlight the clinical dilemmas and problems that may be encountered in clinical practice. Questions are posed to test the reader's thinking, with suggested answers detailed directly beneath each case study or answered within the text.

Enteral nutrition

Case study 1

Percutaneous endoscopic gastrostomy migration

A 45-year-old gentleman with tetraplegia resulting from an accident was admitted to a medical ward with pneumonia. He was reliant upon percutaneous endoscopic gastrostomy (PEG) to meet all his nutritional and fluid requirements. Forty-eight hours following admission, he was referred to the nutrition nurse specialist (NNS) with inflammation around his PEG.

Question 1

Identify two possible causes of inflammation around a PEG tube

---

The triangular external fixation device appeared to be resting against the abdominal wall, but only approximately 10 cm of the PEG tube was visible outside the patient's abdomen. The fixation device was released and removed revealing the 12 cm tube marking.

Question 2

If a PEG tube is positioned correctly, what centimetre (cm) marking would you expect to see at the patient's abdomen?

A gentle pull was exerted on the PEG releasing a further 6 cm of tube from the patient's stomach before resistance was felt, indicating that the internal fixation device was positioned against the stomach wall.

Nursing staff reported that the patient often requested that the position of the fixation device be altered, particularly when his position was changed from lying to sitting. He remained adamant that the fixation plate should not be placed tightly against his abdomen, as he felt that it was responsible for the inflammation around his tube. Nursing staff had been complying with his requests over a period of months, during which time the inflammation had become widespread, a small granuloma had developed and the site had become infected, necessitating a course of antibiotic therapy. Antibiotics successfully treated the infection but the inflammation and granuloma remained.

Question 3

What would be your next course of action?

The need to minimise the movement of the PEG was discussed with the patient and the nursing staff. A practical teaching session was undertaken on the ward, including the patient, to demonstrate the correct positioning of the fixation plate and the effect of poor positioning. With his agreement, following the teaching session a foam dressing was placed around the stoma and the fixation plate repositioned closer to the abdomen. Within a week, the inflammation and size of the granuloma had reduced. In just under four weeks, the site had healed completely.

Answers

Question 1: Identify two possible causes of inflammation around a PEG tube

The most common causes of inflammation around a gastrostomy tube include:

- the external fixation plate being positioned too tightly to the abdomen, causing inflammation that, if left unchecked, will lead to ulceration. This may also be a problem following the insertion of a PEG into a patient who is dehydrated. If the fixation plate is positioned close to the abdomen following the procedure, once the patient starts to receive fluid their tissues will re-perfuse, making the fixation plate dig into the abdomen. Its position should be checked daily and repositioned if necessary to avoid this problem.

- tube migration caused by the external fixation plate being positioned too loosely, allowing the PEG to move excessively in and out of the stoma tract.
- peristomal infection.

Question 2: If a PEG tube is positioned correctly, what centimetre (cm) marking would you expect to see at the patient's abdomen?

Depending on the amount of adipose tissue at the abdomen, it is usual to see from the 2 cm to the 6 cm marker at the entrance to the stoma tract if the tube is correctly positioned and the internal bumper is sitting against the gastric mucosa.

Question 3: What would be your next course of action?

The next course of action should be to discuss with the patient the rationale for advising that the fixation plate be placed close to his abdomen, i.e. the need to minimise unnecessary movement of the PEG in and out of the stoma.

The issue was discussed with the patient and the nursing staff. A practical teaching session was undertaken on the ward, including the patient, to demonstrate correct positioning of the fixation plate and the effect of poor positioning. With his agreement, following the teaching session a foam dressing was placed around the stoma and the fixation plate repositioned closer to the abdomen. Within a week, the inflammation and size of the granuloma had reduced. After almost four weeks, the site had healed completely.

Case study 2

Percutaneous endoscopic gastrostomy stoma development

A 52-year-old lady with motor neurone disease was referred to the Nutrition Support Team (NST) for the insertion of a PEG tube. She attended the endoscopy department as a day case and, following the insertion of the PEG, was discharged home to be followed up the next day.

Her husband was taught how to administer feed and fluid and care for the tube whilst his wife was in hospital and was observed starting a feed and flushing the PEG at home.

Five days following insertion, the husband contacted the NST as he was concerned that the PEG tube had disappeared into the stomach and may be falling out.

Question 1

What may have caused this problem?

The NNS visited the patient at home to discover that the fixation device had been released by a visiting healthcare professional within two days following the insertion of the tube. They had done this to facilitate cleaning around the PEG site. The healthcare professional, feeling a 'pull' on the PEG, had loosened the fixation plate to prevent any discomfort.

Answer

Question 1: What may have caused this problem?

By releasing the fixation device within the first 48 hours of insertion, the 'pull' felt was the stomach moving away from the internal abdominal wall. As the positioning was not corrected in the following three days, the formation of a tract took a further four weeks to fully develop.

(NB: It is worth noting that in both of these case studies the gastrostomy tube had been allowed to migrate into the stomach. In so doing, not only was the patient at increased risk of mechanical irritation but, more importantly, the internal fixation device could have obstructed the pylorus, causing outflow obstruction of feed and gastric contents and probable admission to hospital.)

Case study 3

Buried bumper

A 78-year-old parkinsonian man was referred with decreasing oral intake. His swallow had gradually deteriorated over some time and, following a speech and language therapist's assessment, it was agreed that a PEG would be required to provide long-term access for enteral nutrition and a secure means of administering his medication.

His wife was his main carer and was taught how to care for the tube and feed administration whilst her husband was in hospital. By the date of discharge, she felt confident she could manage to care for the PEG and administer the feed at home. The district nurses were asked to visit weekly to advance and rotate the tube. Follow-up was arranged with the NNS and dietitian three times a year.

Ten months following discharge, the NNS was asked to see the patient as the district nurse was unable to advance the PEG tube. The patient was reviewed by the NNS with the district nurse present. At the first attempt, the NNS was unable to move the tube; however, with lubrication the PEG was advanced into the abdomen and rotated. Having seen the PEG move, the district nurse was happy to continue with weekly checks.

Three months later, the patient was referred back to the NNS for the same problem. On review, the NNS was unable to advance the PEG with or without lubrication. The patient was complaining of discomfort on administration of flushes but not the feed, and his wife reported that she was finding it increasingly difficult to flush the tube using a syringe.

Question 1

What is the likely problem here, and what would be the management?

As the tube could not be manipulated, the patient was referred for endoscopy with a suspected buried bumper.

Question 2

How does a 'buried bumper' arise and how can it be prevented?

Endoscopy showed that the internal bumper was completely buried in the gastric mucosa and could only be detected by administering a water flush through the PEG during the procedure. It was not possible to free the PEG, and so to maintain access to provide the patient's nutrition a second PEG was inserted and a surgical opinion was sought for removal of the original PEG.

Question 3

What options are there for PEG removal and which would you choose here?

In view of the comorbidity of the patient, a minimal approach was adopted to remove the PEG: it was cut off at the level of the abdomen and the site covered with a sterile transparent dressing.

Within a week, the site of the first PEG was infected and a small but continual flow of gastric fluid was leaking out of the PEG stump. This was not improved with a course of antibiotics. The patient was admitted back to hospital for a laparotomy and removal of PEG stump. Once removed, the site of the old PEG healed. There were no further problems with the second PEG.

Answers

Question 1: What is the likely problem here, and what would be the management?

This is clearly a case of a buried bumper.

Some patients may tense their abdominal muscles expecting some discomfort when their PEG is touched or may not like the sight or feel of anyone touching their PEG. This may cause some resistance when attempts are made to advance and rotate a PEG tube. The use of lubrication at the PEG site or distracting the patient by chatting to them may relax the muscles and facilitate easier movement of the PEG. However, if it feels as though the PEG tube is folding in upon itself and there are reports of increasing difficulty flushing the PEG tube, the likelihood is that the patient has a buried bumper and should be referred back to the NST or for investigation, particularly if the PEG is the patient's only way of receiving nutrition.

Question 2: How does a 'buried bumper' arise and how can it be prevented?

Buried bumper occurs when the internal bumper of the PEG is pressured tightly against the skin. If the position of the bumper is not changed over time, gastric mucosa begins to grow over the bumper, encasing it and eventually covering it completely, i.e. burying it. Therefore, at endoscopy, the bumper may not be seen but may only be identified by:

- the administration of a water flush from the external end of the PEG tube
- observation of movement of the gastric mucosa on external manipulation of the PEG tube.

Question 3: What options are there for PEG removal and which would you choose here?

There are two options for removal of a PEG tube with a buried bumper:

- surgical excision

- conservative management: cutting the PEG tube as close to the abdomen as possible and sealing with a transparent dressing until the mucosal overgrowth covers the internal bumper completely sealing the lumen and external granulation covers the PEG stump. This is effective in some patients but as can be seen from above may be prone to infection.

This case study highlights the importance of advancing and rotating a PEG tube regularly following the development of the stoma tract. In our experience, nurses will often report that the PEG tube is regularly rotated but, without advancing the PEG into the stomach, rotating is of little benefit in preventing a buried bumper.

Case study 4

Gastric or jejunal feeding

A 59-year-old man was admitted with a subdural haematoma. He made an incomplete recovery, necessitating transfer to a nursing home with a PEG to meet his fluid and nutritional needs upon his discharge.

Two weeks following his transfer, nursing staff reported regular bouts of vomiting following the administration of feed. Nurses were asked to monitor his bowels for constipation. One week later, they reported that he was still vomiting but that constipation was not an issue.

Question 1

What other issues may cause vomiting during PEG feeding?

A trial of the antiemetic metoclopramide was commenced but was discontinued after a two-week period as the patient was unable to tolerate it. Three weeks later, the patient was admitted to hospital with dehydration and weight loss. Following consultation with the NST, a decision was made to insert a jejunal extension through the current PEG tube, giving him a percutaneous gastrojejunostomy (PEGJ).

The jejunal extension was inserted uneventfully with endoscopic assistance. The nurse accompanying the patient was shown how to care for the tube and written instructions were provided for continuing care of the tube in the nursing home.

Four months later, a home visit was carried out to review the patient. No further vomiting had occurred and he had started to gain weight.

Ten months later, he was re-referred to the NST with vomiting and weight loss.

Question 2

Consider the possible causes of this.

He was reviewed by the NNS and dietitian. At external examination of the feeding tube, no jejunal extension was seen or felt. The correct attachments remained in place at the end of the feeding tube but there was no jejunal extension connected to them. The nursing staff reported that the patient had passed a long thin tube rectally two months previously. Unfortunately, this had not been reported to any healthcare professional outside of the nursing home.

The patient had also started to vomit again at about this time.

The patient was admitted as a day case for insertion of a second jejunal extension.

Training sessions were provided for all levels of nursing staff regarding care of the tube and when to report problems. Six months later, there were no further problems with vomiting.

Answers

Question 1: What other issues may cause vomiting during PEG feeding?

Common causes of vomiting during PEG feeding include:

- the rate of feed being administered is too high
- the feed is administered at too cold a temperature
- gastric stasis.

Question 2: Consider the possible causes of this.

Vomiting and weight loss at this point may be due to:

- the PEGJ extension becoming dislodged
- the PEG/PEGJ extension could be partially obstructing the gastric outlet
- the feed may have been altered and poorly tolerated.

Other possible causes include:

- underlying infection
- extension of his head injury.

Case study 5

Spontaneous expulsion of a gastrostomy tube

A 26-year-old man with cerebral palsy presented with worsening dysphagia. He was referred to the NST for consideration of his nutritional needs. As he had lost over 7 kg in weight and his nutritional intake consisted of a couple of teaspoons of yoghurt and sips of thickened fluid, it was decided to insert a PEG. Following PEG insertion, the patient started to gain weight and was able to be discharged home. There were no problems identified with enteral feeding at review for the first 18 months following discharge.

Two weeks after review, the patient presented to his general practitioner with a four-day history of vomiting and showed signs of abdominal discomfort, particularly during the administration of feed or fluids. The GP recommended stopping the feed and referred the patient to a district general hospital for consideration of an underlying abscess. However, before the patient could be seen, he attended the accident and emergency department of his local hospital as an emergency as he had spontaneously expelled his PEG tube out of his abdomen in one piece. A balloon gastrostomy was inserted through the stoma by the on-call gastroenterologist and the patient was discharged home.

His carers were taught how to care for this new tube and the district nurse was asked to check the balloon on a weekly basis. However, the patient expelled the gastrostomy within three weeks. Over the next two months, the patient expelled a further three balloon gastrostomy tubes, each with a burst balloon. However, as the patient's family was unwilling to put him through another endoscopy, the decision was made to persevere with a balloon gastrostomy.

Two weeks later, the patient was admitted overnight with vomiting and abdominal pain and a severe acid burn from gastric leakage around the gastrostomy site. Endoscopy was advised. It showed the balloon had become lodged in the pylorus. The gastrostomy was repositioned and the patient discharged home with a proton pump inhibitor (PPI) for gastric acid suppression.

Question 1

What possible causes are there for the continued vomiting, and how would you manage them?

Five days later, the gastrostomy was expelled following a bout of vomiting. The patient was reviewed by the NNS. It appeared that vomiting commonly occurred when the patient was moved by carers in the morning during washing and dressing activities and when getting out of bed. The acid burn around the PEG appeared to be improving but had not healed completely.

Answer

Question 1: What possible causes are there for the continued vomiting, and how would you manage them?

Two possible causes were identified:

* The patient had an overnight feed followed by immediate administration of medication through the gastrostomy. The feed was stopped 30 minutes prior to carers getting him out of bed.
* The PPI (Lansoprazole) was administered directly following a feed. The prescription read 'give in the morning' but was being given immediately following the administration of an overnight feed into an already full stomach.

The management plan agreed with the carers included starting the feed earlier in the evening and finishing earlier in the morning. This enabled the patient to have a break from the feed before the carers began moving him. The timing of the PPI was changed so that it could be administered in the evening, when the stomach was empty.

A two-week trial of metoclopramide was commenced to assist gastric emptying.

As a result, the patient experienced no further vomiting, the acid burn around the gastrostomy site healed and the balloon gastrostomy remained in situ for five months before being replaced.

Case study 6

Administration of medication through a PEG

A 49-year-old lady was admitted with nausea and vomiting. She had known spina bifida, chronic back pain, fluctuating swallowing abilities and ulcerative colitis, for which she had an ileostomy. She had a PEG in situ and at the time of admission was unable to take any fluids orally.

Her carer crushed each of her medicines in the same container, administered them as a single dose via the PEG with one 50 ml flush of water on completion. Not surprisingly, the carer reported that the PEG was prone to blocking.

Her medication was as follows:

- citalopram: 20 mg tablet once daily
- morphine: 100 mg capsule twice daily
- temazepam: 10 mg tablet at night
- omeprazole: 20 mg capsule in the morning
- methicillin-resistant Staphylococcus aureus (MRSA): topical treatment
- multivitamin: one tablet a day
- paracetamol dispersible: two tablets four times per day
- enoxaparin: 40 mg subcutaneously daily.

Question 1

How could these medications be changed to make it easier to give via PEG?

The citalopram, morphine, temazepam and multivitamins could all be given as drops or liquids. **(NB: the dose of citalopram needs to be converted: 20 mg tablet = 16 mg liquid.)**

While an in-patient, it was observed that she regurgitated enteral feed.

Question 2

How could this be helped?

It was arranged for her to have a jejunal extension inserted through her PEG.

At the time of endoscopy, it was noted that she had gastritis, and the gastroenterologist performing the endoscopy prescribed sucralfate.

Question 3

What are the potential problems with the administration of this drug for this patient?

Sucralfate needs to be taken orally and therefore would not work if given via the PEGJ. A bezoar (a relatively insoluble complex) forms between the protein in the enteral feeds and the aluminium from the antacids or sucralfate (sucralfate is about 18% aluminium) (Tomlin & Dixon, 1996).

She then contracted a urinary tract infection which required treatment with ciprofloxacin.

Question 4

Do you know of any problems associated with the administration of ciprofloxacin?

The pharmacist on the NST arranged with the dietitian for her feeds to be given intermittently as ciprofloxacin needs to be delivered to an empty stomach for absorption.

Studies have shown that the bioavailability and serum levels of ciprofloxacin may be reduced by up to 30% with enteral feeds (Noer & Angaran, 1990).

Answers

Question 1: How could these medications be changed to make it easier to give via PEG?

It would be sensible to contact the pharmacist to see whether any of these medications could be changed to liquid preparations. For example, the citalopram, morphine capsules, temazepam tablets, and multivitamins could all be given as drops or liquids.

Question 2: How could this be helped?

There are a number of measures that could be introduced to reduce reflux and regurgitation of feed:

- Look at the positioning of the patient during feeds. Sitting the patient as upright as possible is recommended.
- Check at what the rate the feed is being administered. It may need to be reduced. Liaise with the patient's dietitian.
- Monitor and record the level of additional fluid the patient is receiving in addition to the feed (e.g. with medication). The patient's overall fluid intake may need to be reduced.
- Monitor bowel movements: constipation may exacerbate gastrointestinal symptoms.
- Where these measures are unsuccessful, the placement of a jejunal extension through the PEG may need to be considered – making the feeding tube a PEGJ (percutaneous endoscopic gastrojejunostomy).

In the case of this lady, a jejunal extension was inserted through her PEG.

Question 3: What are the potential problems with the administration of this drug for this patient?

Sucralfate is used to treat chronic gastritis, gastrointestinal ulcers and in the prevention of gastrointestinal bleeding. For it to be effective, it needs to be taken orally so that it passes through the stomach. If administered through the PEGJ, it would bypass the stomach and would therefore be ineffective in treating this patient's gastritis. If given via the PEGJ, it combines with protein in the enteral feed, and the aluminium from the antacids or sucralfate form an insoluble bond (Tomlin & Dixon, 1996) blocking the feeding tube.

Question 4: Do you know of any problems associated with the administration of ciprofloxacin?

Ciprofloxacin needs to be delivered to an empty stomach for absorption. Therefore, the pharmacist on the NST had to liaise with the patient's dietitian to arrange for her feeds to be given intermittently until the course of ciprofloxacin had been completed.

Combined enteral/parenteral nutrition

Case study 1

Providing nutrition via the appropriate route

An 85-year-old gentleman with known chronic obstructive pulmonary disease (COPD) was admitted with pneumonia. He was found to have dysphagia, confirmed by a speech and language assessment, and was malnourished. Owing to his poor nutritional state and dysphagia, he was taking longer to recover from his pneumonia. However, as his swallow was unsafe he was made nil by mouth (NBM) and was referred for nutrition support.

Question 1

What methods of nutrition support are available and which would you choose here?

It was elected to pass a nasogastric (NG) tube and use this for enteral feeding until he had recovered from his pneumonia. Then he would be reassessed to establish whether he was at long-term risk of aspiration and therefore required a longer-term method of nutrition support, such as a PEG.

Unfortunately, it was not possible to pass the NG tube, either by the ward nursing team, medical staff or the ear, nose and throat team.

Question 2

Consider what action you would take in this situation.

The patient was referred to the NST for consideration of his nutritional needs. Owing to his breathing difficulties, it was felt that it would be risky to attempt insertion of a gastrostomy at this stage. He was assessed by the NST, who agreed to provide parenteral nutrition (PN) until his condition stabilised; however, no central catheter access was present at that time.

Question 3

What routes are available for PN provision and which would be most suitable here?

This gentleman was unable to lie flat, owing to his pneumonia; so the decision was made to insert a PICC (peripherally inserted central catheter) to ensure central access. PN was then provided.

Four days later, the patient was reassessed by the speech and language team, who found that his swallow had improved sufficiently to allow him to start to take some oral diet, but it was acknowledged that this would be compromised by his associated breathlessness.

Oral intake was recommenced and PN discontinued. However, following recovery from his pneumonia, his oral intake did not improve sufficiently to prevent him from losing further weight.

Question 4

What would you do now?

Oral diet was supplemented with sip feeds but his intake continued to be limited by his breathlessness. A decision was made that, to ensure his nutritional status over the long term, a PEG or a radiologically inserted gastrostomy (RIG) should be inserted when his respiratory status stabilised sufficiently to allow the procedure to take place. Within five days, he was stable enough to have a PEG inserted. Following the procedure, this gentleman continued to take the foods he enjoyed orally but his remaining fluid and nutritional requirements were provided via the PEG tube. Three weeks following insertion of the PEG, the patient had gained two kilograms in weight and had recovered sufficiently from his pneumonia to enable him to go home with support.

Answers

Question 1: What methods of nutrition support are available and which would you choose here?

Enteral nutrition: nasogastric feeding – the short-term option. Long-term options include gastrostomy feeding or jejunal feeding.

For this patient, nasogastric feeding would be the first option of choice. Parenteral feeding options: peripheral or central line feeding. Not the option of choice at this stage as this patient had a functional gastrointestinal tract.

Question 2: Consider what action you would take in this situation.

It was not possible to insert a nasogastric tube, the patient was not fit enough to undergo insertion of a PEG or RIG. His nutritional status was already compromised and it was felt that without intervention his recovery from pneumonia would be prolonged. PN was provided on the basis that enteral nutrition would commence as soon as possible and that a gastrostomy would be inserted for meeting the patient's long-term nutritional requirements.

Question 3: What routes are available for PN provision and which would be most suitable here?

PN may be given centrally using a dedicated lumen of a central line, or by a PICC. Alternatively, a peripheral cannula can be used in the short term with selected formulations of PN.

Question 4: What would you do now?

The aim of treatment here is to stop this patient from losing weight using the gastrointestinal tract rather than the intravenous route. The first step would be to supplement his oral diet and use sip feeds between meals.

Unfortunately, this patient's oral intake continued to be limited by his breathlessness.

Parenteral nutrition

Case study 1

Appropriate use of PN?

A 50-year-old lady was referred to the NST for PN with a diagnosis of small bowel obstruction. Earlier in the year, an adenocarcinoma had been found by chance within a uterine fibroid at hysterectomy. She had subsequently developed a colovaginal fistula and required a defunctioning colostomy. She then had six cycles of chemotherapy. Following this, she developed small bowel obstruction.

At laparotomy, peritoneal seedlings were identified along with an ileo-caecal mass, which it was found difficult to remove surgically. Thus, all further treatment was with non-curative intent.

Following surgery, the patient developed an abdominal wall abscess requiring debridement and drainage on two occasions.

She then went home for convalescence.

Two weeks later, she was admitted with abdominal pain and was found to have small bowel fistulae. She required further surgery with debridement and drainage.

Following surgery the patient was referred for PN as she was NBM. It was 20th December and she was planning to go home for Christmas. She had no central access. Medical staff reported that it would not be possible to provide central access for another 24 hours.

Question 1

Would you start PN in this lady?

Once central access was provided, PN was started, but three days later the patient refused venepuncture as she had been informed that morning that all treatment provided to her was palliative. She had been encouraged to refuse any procedure she did not want, and so no blood results were available to calculate her electrolyte requirements in the PN.

Question 2

How would you handle PN provision under these circumstances?

Question 3

Would you continue PN?

The PN was stopped and enteral feeding was attempted with a low-residue diet. On Christmas Eve, the patient was transferred to a hospice on a low-residue diet; she died soon after.

Answers

Question 1: Would you start PN in this lady?

This is a controversial case where the use of PN has no immediately obvious timespan, and therefore it may have been inappropriate to start it. However, given that she had significantly little gut available for nutritional use, it was felt reasonable at the time to use PN until her problems could be surgically corrected.

Question 2: How would you handle PN provision under these circumstances?

If monitoring of her biochemistry was not possible, PN cannot be provided safely, particularly as she was likely to have abnormal biochemistry with her ongoing small- and large-bowel problems, sepsis and possible renal impairment. Under these circumstances, she should be counselled as to the consequences of refusing phlebotomy (which could take place via her central access) and PN withdrawn if she could not be monitored.

Question 3: Would you continue PN?

As monitoring was refused, PN was withdrawn and possible enteral alternatives were considered. An elemental diet was considered as she had some small-bowel bioavailable, but was considered inappropriate in view of its poor palatability and her condition. A low-residue diet was started as this allowed freedom to leave hospital: her main goal.

Case study 2

Identifying the source of infection

A 45-year-old woman admitted with small-bowel obstruction was managed on the intensive-care unit. She had an existing multi-lumen jugular central line, which had been inserted three days earlier, with an unused lumen dedicated to PN.

Three days after commencing PN, she developed a high-grade pyrexia. As there was no obvious source of infection, the central line was blamed as the most likely cause and so was removed.

However, the patient's temperature did not resolve.

Question 1

What action should have been taken to identify whether the central line was the source of infection?

Within 48 hours, a single lumen Hickman line was inserted to be used solely for the administration of PN. PN was administered uneventfully over a period of three weeks at which point the patient developed a pyrexia again. Once again, there was no obvious source of infection, and so the central access became the focus of attention. The NST advised that peripheral and central blood cultures were taken, which showed no subsequent growth. The Hickman line remained in situ, and further investigations were undertaken to identify the source of sepsis. An abdominal computerised tomography (CT) scan showed signs in keeping with small-intestinal necrosis and collections of pus. Appropriate treatment was commenced.

Question 2

At this point, what additions could be made to the PN?

Glutamine was added to the PN as the patient was septic and catabolic.

PN was provided for a further four weeks. A trial of oral fluids and supplements was then commenced. As the patient seemed to be tolerating oral intake, PN was stopped after 48 hours and the Hickman line removed. Unfortunately, within three days the patient started vomiting and was able to tolerate less than 500 kcal/day orally.

Question 3

How would you maintain nutrition support at this point?

PN was recommenced and a central line was inserted to facilitate this.

The patient returned to theatre for further bowel surgery and was supported with PN uneventfully for the next eight days. Following this, a trial with oral fluids was commenced, which was well tolerated. The PN was decreased gradually as oral intake increased over a 48-hour period. As oral diet was now established, PN was discontinued.

Answers

Question 1: What action should have been taken to identify whether the central line was the source of infection?

If the patient with a central line presents with a pyrexia where the source cannot be identified, blood cultures should be obtained simultaneously from the central line and from a peripheral vein. Results should show whether the central line is the source of the infection and may prevent needless removal of the line.

Question 2: At this point, what additions could be made to the PN?

The addition of glutamine has been shown to be beneficial under these circumstances (Jiang *et al.*, 1999).

Question 3: How would you maintain nutrition support?

As this patient's gut was not functioning adequately, PN would be the preferable option for nutrition support until function resumes.

Case study 3

Is the line to blame?

A 54-year-old gentleman was admitted with small-bowel obstruction.

He underwent a laparotomy and five days later was referred for nutrition support. He had been NBM since surgery and was for gut rest. He had an existing jugular central line with one unused lumen, which was dedicated to the infusion of PN. Within three days of starting PN, he was pyrexial with no overt focus for infection.

Question 1

What could be the source of infection?

His jugular line was exposed. Nursing staff reported extreme difficulties in keeping a dressing in place for any length of time. The site around the central line had become inflamed, with the patient reporting discomfort on neck movement and administration of fluid. Therefore, the line was removed and sent for culture. Appropriate antibiotics were started and a PICC was inserted for PN. Trials of oral intake of water were commenced at 30 ml/hour gradually increasing to 60 ml/hour.

Six days later, the patient was found to have a high blood glucose, was pyrexial and had a chest infection. He was still unable to tolerate more than 60 ml of fluid orally each hour. Radiological studies showed the presence of an intestinal fistula. All oral intake was stopped but PN continued.

Just over a week later, the patient's condition had improved enough to enable him to start to move around the ward.

Question 2

How would you alter the patient's regimen to give him more freedom to encourage his mobility?

One morning, nursing staff reported that the volumetric pump had kept alarming overnight and that periodically they were finding it difficult to flush the PICC.

Question 3

What could be causing these problems?

Within days, the patient developed a pyrexia with no overt focus for infection. Central and peripheral blood cultures were taken, suggesting that the PICC was the likely source of infection. Therefore, the PICC was removed. Appropriate antibiotics were commenced, following which the patient developed diarrhoea through his stoma. A senior anaesthetist could only obtain IV access in his foot.

Question 4

How might you manage his nutrition now?

After three days, he was vomiting and so PN was required. A Hickman line was inserted. After a further two weeks of PN, trials of oral fluids commenced and the patient was found to be able to tolerate sip feeds.

At this time, the surgical team felt the fistula had healed and had requested that the PN be stopped.

Question 5

How would you advise the surgical team?

As enteral fluid was tolerated, diet was commenced with soup, jelly, ice cream and sip feeds, gradually increasing to a low-fibre diet. As this was well tolerated, PN was stopped. Finally, the Hickman line was removed after he had been eating satisfactorily for three days.

Answers

Question 1: What could be the source of infection?

Jugular lines are often difficult to dress as the central catheter sits close to the hairline and is further disturbed by neck movement and perspiration.

Question 2: How would you alter the patient's regimen to give him more freedom to encourage his mobility?

The rate of PN was increased so that it was administered over 18 hours (as opposed to continuous administration), allowing the patient six hours free of his pump during the day, giving him more freedom to move about.

Question 3: What could be causing these problems?

In this case, the problem was due to a kink that had formed in the PICC under the dressing at the antecubital fossa. Once corrected, nursing staff found flushing easier. The pump, however, continued to alarm periodically. This was attributed to the patient pinching off the lumen as he bent his arm during movement.

Question 4: How might you manage his nutrition now?

Given his repeated problems with access and pyrexia, clearly enteral nutrition was desirable as soon as possible. He was started on a light diet.

Question 5: How would you advise the surgical team?

After receiving PN for a period of over two months, it was advised that enteral feeding should commence slowly and that the PN be gradually reduced until enteral feeding was firmly established.

Case study 4

A case for home PN

A 34-year-old lady with known Crohn's disease presented with a history of nausea and vomiting extending over one week and at the time of admission was unable to tolerate any fluids orally. She reported a gradual loss of weight, of at least two stone (12.7 kg), since the birth of her second child 18 months previously.

She had two young children at home and was experiencing difficulty arranging childcare and was desperate to get home, and was therefore extremely reluctant to be admitted.

Her medical plan on admission included being kept NBM, pending investigations. She was referred to the NST for nutrition advice.

She was assessed by the team, who felt PN was the appropriate option. Insertion of a PICC was arranged and PN commenced.

Question 1

What PN regime would you use?

She was started on a regimen of intravenous vitamins and a 500 kcal bag of PN, as she had not eaten properly in over a week and was thought to be at risk of developing re-feeding syndrome.

On review the following day, the NST found her very tearful, and desperate to get home.

Question 2

How could you manage her PN to facilitate this where possible?

It was explained to her that the PN could be given overnight so that she could go home during the day to be with her family. It was highlighted that administration of fluids overnight would result in urinary frequency, once her level of PN increased, but she was happy to accept this if it gave her the option to spend time at home.

Answers

Question 1: What PN regime would you use?

As this patient had been vomiting for over a week, the risk of developing re-feeding syndrome if her calorific requirements were provided in full immediately would have been high. Therefore, to minimise this risk, she was commenced on IV vitamins and a low-calorie bag of PN. The content of the PN bag would be gradually increased every couple of days in line with biochemistry results until her nutritional requirements were met.

Question 2: How could you manage her PN to facilitate this where possible?

Some larger healthcare organisations have the facilities to offer home PN where the patient can be managed with the support of community services and private PN company facilities. Where this facility is not available, overnight administration of PN in hospital offers the patient some flexibility to remain in their own home during the day.

References

Jiang, Z.M., Cao, J.D., Zhu, X.G. *et al.* (1999) The impact of alanyl-glutamine on clinical safety, nitrogen balance, intestinal permeability and clinical outcome in post operative patients: A randomised, double blind, controlled study of 120 patients. *Journal of Parenteral and Enteral Nutrition* **23** (5), 62–6.

Noer, B.L., Angaran, D.M. (1990) The effect of enteral feedings on ciprofloxacin pharmacokinetics. *Pharmacotherapy* **10**, 254 (Abstract).

Tomlin, M.E., Dixon, S. (1996) Aluminium and nasogastric feeds (a letter). *Pharmaceutical Journal* **256** (40), 44.

Glossary and Abbreviations

adenocarcinoma	a malignant tumour originating in the glandular epithelium
ALP	alkaline phosphatase
ALT	alanine aminotransferase: a liver enzyme that plays a role in protein metabolism; elevated serum levels of ALT are a sign of liver damage from disease or drugs
angular stomatitis	inflammation and fissuring radiating from the commissures of the mouth secondary to predisposing factors such as lost vertical dimension in denture wearers, nutritional deficiencies, atopic dermatitis or candida albicans infection
antecubital fossa	the area in front of the elbow
AST	aspartate aminotransferase
atresia	the absence or closure of a natural passage or channel of the body
atrophy	a wasting-away of a cell, tissue or organ
BANS	British Artificial Nutrition Survey: BANS is a national database of patients receiving artificial nutrition support in the United Kingdom
BAPEN	British Association for Parenteral and Enteral Nutrition
BMI	body mass index: a measure of body weight relative to height used to determine whether people are underweight, at a healthy weight, overweight or obese

BMR	basal metabolic rate: your basal metabolic rate is the minimum calories required to sustain life in a resting individual, i.e. the amount of energy (measured in calories) expended by the body whilst lying asleep in bed all day
bolus feeding	(also known as **intermittent feeding**) the administration of a single delivery of feed through an enteral feeding tube using either a syringe or pump, e.g. 200 ml of feed delivered over a two- to three-minute period; this type of feeding is sometimes used to mimic mealtimes
buried bumper	the migration of the internal bumper of a PEG tube into the gastric or abdominal wall
catabolism	a metabolic process by which organisms are broken down to convert substances into excreted compounds
catecholamine	any of a group of amines derived from catechol that have important physiological effects as neurotransmitters and hormones and include epinephrine, norepinephrine and dopamine
ch	French gauge: this is one of the abbreviations used to describe the internal lumen of a feeding tube
cheilosis	inflammation and cracking of the lips: usually secondary to a vitamin C or B-complex deficiency
coagulopathy	a disease affecting coagulation of the blood
Coeliac disease	atrophy of the villi in the small intestine leading to impaired absorption of nutrients; it is caused by a sensitivity to gluten (a protein found in wheat and rye)
colonisation	the presence, growth and multiplication of an organism without observable clinical symptoms or immune reaction in a patient
colovaginal fistula	a fistula or abnormal connection between the colon and the vagina
CR	controlled release

CRP	C-reactive protein: an antibody found in the blood in certain acute and chronic conditions including infections and cancers; it is a non-specific indicator of inflammation
Dacron cuff	a cuff on a central line which anchors it in position under a tunnel in the skin and prevents it falling out; it also helps protect against infection
defunctioning colostomy	a stoma created to divert faecal flow, so that faeces no longer passes through the anus
delayed cutaneous hypersensitivity (DCH) response	a sensitivity reaction that can take from 24 to 72 hours to develop; mediated by T lymphocytes rather than by antibodies
Diet-induced thermogenesis	the increase in energy expenditure above basal metabolic rate
dysmotility	slow and uncoordinated movement through the gut causing bloating, reflux and nausea
dysphagia	difficulty with swallowing
ECF	extracellular fluid
ECG	electrocardiograph
electrolytes	anions and cations in the blood, tissue fluids and cells, e.g. sodium and potassium
enteropathy	disease of the intestines
erythema	a redness on the surface of the skin due to the congestion of the capillaries
FBC	full blood count
fibrosis	the formation of fibrous tissue
fistula	the development of an abnormal passage between two internal organs or from an internal organ to the body surface
fr	French gauge: this is another option that is used to describe the internal lumen of a feeding tube
gastrojejunostomy tube	a type of enteral feeding tube that is inserted through the abdominal wall into the stomach and through into the jejunum
gastro-oesophageal reflux	the backflow of contents from the stomach into the oesophagus resulting from a relaxation of the lower oesophageal sphincter

gastroparesis	delayed gastric emptying
gastrostomy	an enteral feeding tube inserted through the abdominal wall into the stomach
GI	gastrointestinal
glucagon	a polypeptide hormone secreted by the cells of the islets of Langerhans in response to a fall in blood-sugar levels
gluconeogenesis	synthesis of glucose from non-carbohydrate sources, i.e. proteins and fats; it takes place largely in the liver and serves to maintain blood-glucose levels under conditions of starvation
glutamine	a conditionally essential amino acid required during periods of stress; it is thought to be essential for maintaining intestinal function, immune response and amino acid homeostasis
glycogenolysis	the breaking-down, or catabolism, of the polysaccharide glycogen into molecules of glucose within the body by enzymes
granuloma	an overgrowth of tissue (overgranulation) caused by the increased activity of granulocytes in the epithelial tissue most commonly seen around a gastrostomy tube
GTN	glyceryl trinitrate
hepatomegaly	enlargement of the liver
hypercatabolism	an excessive metabolic breakdown of body tissue, leading to weight loss and wasting
hyperglycaemia	an abnormally raised blood-glucose level
hyperlipidaemia	an abnormally raised blood concentration of lipids
hypertonic	hypertonic solutions contain a high concentration of solute relative to another solution (e.g. the cell's cytoplasm)
hypertriglyceridaemia	an abnormally raised blood concentration of triglycerides
hypoalbuminaemia	an abnormally low concentration of albumin in the blood
hypocaloric	low calorie/low energy
ileus	an obstruction (or temporary paralysis) of the intestines

immunocompromised	the immune system is not functioning normally, because of disease or treatment for disease
inflammatory bowel disease	a term that encompasses both Crohn's disease and ulcerative colitis
inner lumen	the inside of a feeding tube or central catheter
INR	international normalised ratio: this blood test is used to determine the clotting tendency of blood and is used most commonly in conjunction with anticoagulants
intestinal failure	may be due to intestinal obstruction or fistula; may require surgery and prolonged administration of PN
intracellular	within a cell
jejunostomy tube	an enteral tube inserted through the abdominal wall directly into the jejunum for the purpose of nutrition support
LCTs	long-chain triglycerides
LFTs	liver-function tests: used to detect liver damage or disease; combinations of up to five tests are measured at the same time on a blood sample:

- alanine aminotransferase (ALT)
- alkaline phosphatase (ALP)
- aspartate aminotransferase (AST)
- total bilirubin
- albumin
- total protein

lingual papilla	one of numerous projections of the mucous membrane of the dorsum of the tongue
lipid	fat
lipolysis	the breakdown of fat
lumen	the inner cavity or channel of a tube
magenta tongue	purplish-red colouration of the tongue, with oedema and flattening of the filiform papillae, occurring as a result of riboflavin deficiency
malabsorption	impaired absorption of nutrients
MCV	mean corpuscular volume: the average volume of red cells

megaloblastic anaemia	anaemia in which there is a predominant number of megaloblastic erythroblasts, and relatively few normoblasts, among the cells in the bone marrow
micronutrients	essential dietary elements required only in small quantities
motility agent	a medication used to aid the movement of food from the stomach into the intestine
mucocutaneous	relating to or affecting the mucous membrane and the skin
mucositis	inflammation of a mucous membrane
NBM	nil by mouth
NG	nasogastric
NICE	National Institute for Health and Clinical Excellence
NJ	nasojejunal
NPSA	National Patient Safety Agency
NSAIDs	Non-steroidal anti-inflammatory medication, e.g. ibuprofen, diclofenac
nutrition assessment	a comprehensive evaluation to define nutrition status which includes taking a medical history, dietary history, physical examination, anthropometric measurements and laboratory data; usually undertaken by a health professional with skills in nutrition and nutrition support, e.g. a dietitian
nutrition screening	a simple and quick process to detect individuals who are at risk of malnutrition with action points for implementation, e.g. completion of food charts or referral to a dietitian or a speech and language therapist
nutrition support	the provision of nutrients in addition to or as a replacement for normal oral intake, which are administered orally, enterally or parenterally with the aim of improving or maintaining a patient's nutritional status
opiate	a substance, natural or synthetic, that is related in action to morphine and binds to the same, or some of the same, receptors; it is used to treat pain

osmolality	the concentration of osmotically active particles in solution, e.g. enteral feed
outflow obstruction	obstruction to the flow of matter through an organ, e.g. that caused by pyloric stenosis
PEG	percutaneous endoscopic gastrostomy
pH	a symbol relating to the acidity or alkalinity of a solution; a pH of 7 is neutral, above 7 is alkaline and below is acidic
phospholipids	lipids containing one or more phosphate groups, e.g. those derived from glycerol; they are important for the structure and function of cell membranes; they are not stored in large amounts in the body
phytate diet	phytates are found in bran, seeds and grain and are associated with fibre in these foods; phytates bind minerals such as calcium, iron, magnesium and zinc, and can therefore contribute to mineral deficiencies in individuals with a high-phytate and low-mineral intake
platelet aggregation	the attachment of platelets to one another; this clumping together can be induced by a number of agents (e.g. thrombin, collagen) and is part of the mechanism leading to the formation of a thrombus
PN	parenteral nutrition: the provision of nutrition support through intravenous administration of nutrients such as amino acids, glucose, fat, electrolytes, vitamins and trace elements
poikilothermic	having a varying body temperature
PPI	proton pump inhibitor: a type of drug used to heal gastric and duodenal ulcers
proteolysis	the hydrolytic breakdown of proteins into simpler, soluble substances, such as peptides and amino acids; occurs during digestion
QDS	four times a day: regularly used abbreviation on a prescription

Quetelet's index	(or body mass index) is a statistical measure of the weight of a person scaled according to height; it was invented between 1830 and 1850 by the Belgian polymath Adolphe Quetelet
radiation enteritis	a functional disorder of the large and small bowel that occurs during or following a course of radiation therapy to the abdomen, pelvis or rectum
rhinitis	inflammation of the mucous membrane of the nose
Ryle's tube	a wide-bore PVC nasogastric tube used for the aspiration of gastric contents
Schofield equation	a method of estimating the BMR in calories of adult men and women
scleroderma	an autoimmune disease affecting blood vessels and collagen production, resulting in hardening of the skin
sequelae	the plural of 'sequela', which is the medical term for 'consequence': a condition that follows the occurrence of disease; used especially of diseases or other morbid conditions resulting from the preceding disease
short bowel syndrome	a malabsorption syndrome resulting from extensive re-section of the small intestine
SR	sustained release
tannins	naturally occurring in plant polyphenols, their main characteristic is they bind and precipitate proteins; commonly found in tea and red wine, they have antioxidant activity (tannins, particularly those in tea, have the less desirable effect of binding with iron to inhibit its absorption)
tetraplegia	otherwise known as quadriplegia: a paralysis of all four limbs, both arms and both legs; may be as a result of a high spinal cord accident or stroke
thrombophlebitis	inflammation of a vein
thrombosis	the development or presence of a thrombus
transdermal	entering through the dermis, or skin: a method of administering medication, e.g. in the form of a patch or ointment

total protein	measures albumin and all other proteins in blood, including antibodies
trace elements	a group of chemicals that, in very small quantities, are essential to the body's appropriate functioning, growth and development
transferrin	a protein that carries iron in the bloodstream
U & Es	urea and electrolytes: a commonly requested blood test
volumetric pump	a pump that accurately measures the volume of fluid administered through it; essential to the administration of PN
WCC	white blood cell count
Wernicke's encephalopathy	a severe syndrome caused by an inadequate intake or absorption of thiamine (vitamin B)
xerophthalmia	a dryness of the conjunctiva and cornea owing to vitamin A deficiency
xiphoid process	the lowest point of the sternum; also known as the xiphisternum

Index

Abbreviations: CVC, central venous catheter; NJ, nasojejunal; NNS, nutrition nurse specialist; NS, nutrition support; NST, Nutrition Support Team; PEAT, Patient Environment Action Team; PEG, percutaneous endoscopic gastrostomy; PEGJ, percutaneous endoscopic gastrojejunostomy; PN, parenteral nutrition; RIG, radiologically inserted gastrostomy.